What To Eat
When You're
Pregnant
and Vegetarian

PEARSON

At Pearson, we believe in learning – all kinds of learning for all kinds of people. Whether it's at home, in the classroom or in the workplace, learning is the key to improving our life chances.

That's why we're working with leading authors to bring you the latest thinking and the best practices, so you can get better at the things that are important to you. You can learn on the page or on the move, and with content that's always crafted to help you understand quickly and apply what you've learned.

If you want to upgrade your personal skills or accelerate your career, become a more effective leader or more powerful communicator, discover new opportunities or simply find more inspiration, we can help you make progress in your work and life.

Pearson is the world's leading learning company. Our portfolio includes the Financial Times, Penguin, Dorling Kindersley, and our educational business, Pearson International.

Every day our work helps learning flourish, and wherever learning flourishes, so do people.

To learn more please visit us at: **www.pearson.com/uk**

What To Eat
When You're
Pregnant
and Vegetarian

The complete guide to healthy eating

Dr Rana Conway

Harlow, England • London • New York • Boston • San Francisco • Toronto • Sydney • Auckland • Singapore • Hong Kong
Tokyo • Seoul • Taipei • New Delhi • Cape Town • São Paulo • Mexico City • Madrid • Amsterdam • Munich • Paris • Milan

PEARSON EDUCATION LIMITED
Edinburgh Gate
Harlow CM20 2JE
United Kingdom
Tel: +44 (0)1279 623623
Web: www.pearson.com/uk

First published 2013 (print and electronic)

Pearson Education is not responsible for the content of third-party internet sites.

ISBN: 978-0-273-78577-4 (print)
        978-0-273-78872-0 (PDF)
        978-0-273-78871-3 (ePub)

British Library Cataloguing-in-Publication Data
A catalogue record for the print edition is available from the British Library

Library of Congress Cataloging-in-Publication Data
Conway, Rana.
  What to eat when you're pregnant and vegetarian : the complete guide to healthy eating / Dr. Rana Conway.
    pages cm
  Includes index.
  ISBN 978-0-273-78577-4 (print) -- ISBN 978-0-273-78872-0 (pdf) -- ISBN 978-0-273-78871-3 (epub)
  1. Pregnancy--Nutritional aspects. 2. Vegetarianism. 3. Mothers--Nutrition. 4. Prenatal care. I. Title.
  RG559.C664 2013
  618.2'42--dc23
                        2013011276

Contains public sector information licensed under the Open Government Licence (OGL) v1.0. www.nationalarchives.gov.uk/doc/open-government-licence.

The vegetarian eatwell plate on page 34 is published courtesy of the Vegetarian Society, www.vegsoc.org.

10 9 8 7 6 5 4 3 2 1
17 16 15 14 13

Front cover image © Nacivet/Getty Images
Text design by Design Deluxe

Print edition typeset in 9.5/13pt Neo Sans Std by 30
Printed in Great Britain by Henry Ling Ltd., at the Dorset Press, Dorchester, Dorset

NOTE THAT ANY PAGE CROSS REFERENCES REFER TO THE PRINT EDITION

To my three beautiful babies –
Joseph, Daniel and Madeleine

Contents

About the author

Rana Conway is a registered nutritionist and a member of the Nutrition Society. Over the past 20 years she has established herself as an expert in nutrition for pregnancy and childhood. She has worked at leading universities and first researched the diets of pregnant vegetarians for her PhD, which she was awarded in 1997. She is *Practical Parenting and Pregnancy* magazine's nutrition expert and has written three books: *Meals Without Tears: How to Get Your Child to Eat Healthily and Happily* (Pearson, 2007), *What To Eat When You're Pregnant: Including the A–Z of What's Safe and What's Not* (Pearson, 2nd edition 2011) and *Weaning Made Easy* (White Ladder, 2011). She lives in London with her husband and three children.

Acknowledgements

A big thank you to everyone who provided me with help, advice and encouragement in writing this book: Samantha Jackson, Lucy Carter, Rachael Stock, Emma Shackleton, Emma Devlin, Jane Graham Maw, Jennifer Christie, Patrick Bonham, Cherry Poussa, Professor Philip Calder (University of Southampton), Dr Adrienne Cullum (NICE), Adam Hardgrave and Olu Adetokunbo (Food Standards Agency), Iain Gillespie (Health Protection Agency), Deb Futers (South Staffordshire PCT), Fiona Ford (Centre for Pregnancy Nutrition, University of Sheffield), Sandra Hood, Amanda Baker and Verity Hunt-Shepperd (Vegan Society), Liz O'Neill and Su Taylor (Vegetarian Society), Lorraine Hughes and Carol Key (Sainsbury's), Abigail Enaburekhan (Tesco), Jaqueline Newson (Higher Nature), Lucy Balaam (Vitabiotics), Tracey Cope (Cauldron Foods), Rob Bookham (Bookhams) and Heather Davies (Kellogg). Thank you also to the Healthy Start team at the Department of Health, Tommy's, Vegusto and Bute Island Foods Ltd. Lastly, thank you to Olly Conway (editorial, computer and emotional support, and husband).

1 How to have a healthy vegetarian pregnancy

Healthy eating is never more important than when you are pregnant. Your diet will affect you and your baby, now and for years to come. It can even influence your grandchildren's health. In the immediate term, a healthy diet can help prevent constipation and other common pregnancy problems. It will also provide the energy and nutrients your baby needs to grow and develop in the coming months, so he or she has the best start in life. What you eat in pregnancy is also important for your baby's long-term health, including the risk of allergies and heart disease.

During pregnancy, your diet needs to supply all your normal energy and nutrient requirements, but it also has to:

- provide all the needs of your growing baby;
- fuel the growth of new tissue, including breasts, uterus and placenta;
- lay down a store for the final weeks of pregnancy when your baby is growing rapidly, and for breastfeeding.

You probably already know that being a vegetarian provides many advantages to health, including lower risks of obesity, heart disease, type 2 diabetes and certain types of cancer. However, sometimes vegetarians, or perhaps more often their relatives, have doubts about whether a vegetarian diet is ideal for pregnancy. You can reassure anyone with concerns that expert groups including the NHS and the British Medical Association (BMA) have reviewed the evidence and concluded that well-planned vegetarian diets can meet all the requirements you and your baby have. Studies carried out in the UK and US have found no differences between the birth weights of babies born to lacto-ovo-vegetarians and meat-eaters. Researchers looking at vegans living in a commune in Tennessee also found completely normal birth weights. It should, however, be pointed out that the commune members took multivitamin and mineral supplements and received advice about increasing protein intake. This shows that no animal products are necessary to make a healthy baby when women plan their diet carefully and take appropriate supplements.

Having a well-planned diet is vital for all pregnant women, and in many ways vegetarian diets are healthier than those of meat-eaters. They are more likely to meet the government's five-a-day target, to include enough fibre and not to have too much saturated fat. However, as a vegetarian you need to make more effort to ensure a good intake of certain nutrients, including omega 3s and vitamin D. If you're a vegan you also need to be particularly careful about getting enough calcium and vitamin B_{12}.

If you're feeling bombarded with information about what you should and shouldn't eat it can be confusing, especially if you get conflicting advice. The most reliable and up-to-date guidelines come from the Food Standards Agency (FSA), the Department of Health, the National Institute for Clinical Excellence (NICE) and the NHS. Their advice is often referred to by other organisations such as the Royal College of Midwives, the British Nutrition Foundation and the NCT (formerly the National Childbirth Trust). If you get advice from your doctor or midwife that goes against official guidelines, bear in mind they may be slightly out of date rather than there really being a difference of opinion. Be careful about taking advice from unqualified individuals online. Internet forums can provide valuable support and a sense of camaraderie, but just because someone ate Brie throughout their pregnancy and had a healthy 9lb baby it doesn't mean there isn't any risk in doing the same. Such messages may be well meant but they don't prove anything - some smokers live to be 100. It is much better to follow advice based on research studies as this reflects the experiences of large numbers of women.

What being a 'vegetarian' means
Throughout this book the word **vegetarian** is used to include **vegans**, who don't eat any animal products, and **lacto-ovo-vegetarians**, who include milk and eggs in their diet.

Early learning

What you eat now can affect your baby for life. The nutrition a baby receives in the womb affects how he or she grows, and this in turn affects the chances of becoming obese in the future, and of developing high blood pressure, type 2 diabetes, heart disease and some cancers. For several decades researchers have known that the health of adults is related to their birth weight and placental weight (which also reflects a mother's nutrient supply). They are now beginning to discover how this happens and why smaller babies are at greater risk of degenerative diseases in later life. It is believed that babies are somehow 'programmed' in the womb. It seems that if they are malnourished their overall growth suffers and so does the development of their vital organs such as the heart and kidneys, putting them at increased risk of poor health in later life. For example, it has been found that some babies are born with half as many nephrons in their kidneys as others, which means they are less able to cope with salt, and more likely to get high blood pressure.

Poor diet in the womb doesn't mean a baby is doomed, but it makes them more vulnerable. They are less resilient to the effects of salt, saturated fat, alcohol and other hazards in modern life, such as stress and a lack of exercise. Part of the problem is that there is often a mismatch between food supply in the womb and diet later on. If babies are under-nourished before birth, their body adapts, ready for a life of food deprivation. If they are then born into an environment where food is actually abundant, their bodies can't cope.

In 2011, research was published showing that what a woman eats during pregnancy can actually affect her baby's DNA. It was found that eating a low-carbohydrate diet in early pregnancy could result in epigenetic changes – alterations in the way specific genes work, although the genetic sequence remains the same. A small adjustment to a baby's DNA caused by a low carbohydrate diet was found to result in more body fat in childhood. The researchers were surprised at how significant a difference early diet could make. The epigenetic changes due to a low-carbohydrate diet in early pregnancy explained a quarter of the difference in fatness of the children six to nine years later. Other research has shown that epigenetic changes are passed on to future generations. So what you eat now could influence your baby's DNA, which in turn will affect his or her own children's health. This can seem incredibly daunting but eating a healthy diet is relatively simple, as you'll see in the next chapter.

Flavour learning in the womb
The food you eat during pregnancy affects the flavour of the amniotic fluid your baby is swimming in and swallowing. When babies start to have solids, they are more likely to enjoy particular flavours, such as garlic or carrot juice, if their mothers had these in late pregnancy. By eating a wide range of healthy foods now you can increase the chances of your baby doing the same and hopefully avoid fussy eating.

Allergy-proofing your baby

Women with a family history of allergies sometimes avoid certain foods during pregnancy in the hope that this will protect their baby from developing allergies. However, trials where this has been tried have shown that avoiding foods such as peanuts, dairy foods, wheat or eggs during pregnancy is not beneficial. It does not appear to protect a baby from developing allergies and it can mean that both a mother and her baby miss out on vital nutrients. However, there Is some evidence that you may be able to reduce your baby's risk of developing allergies and allergic-type conditions by adjusting your diet in other ways.

A study of more than 2,000 preschool children in the Bristol area looked at the incidence of wheezing and eczema in relation to mineral levels at birth. It was found that these problems were less common among children who were born with higher levels of iron and selenium. So, by getting enough iron and selenium, you could be helping protect your child from some allergies (see pages 96 and 122 to find out where these minerals are found). Research has also found that the risk of asthma may be reduced by eating apples during pregnancy, and eating plenty of citrus fruit and yellow and green vegetables may provide protection against eczema.

The types of fat in your diet may also be important, although research regarding this is in the early stages and isn't conclusive. One study found that having a high ratio of omega 6 to omega 3 fatty acids increased allergy risks, so it is a good idea to look at the balance of dietary fats in your diet and make adjustments if necessary (see page 129). Another study, conducted in Australia, found that pregnant women who took DHA supplements had babies three times less likely to show signs of egg allergy when they were one year old. It had been hoped that the supplements might protect against eczema, and although this wasn't found to be the case, it appeared that eczema symptoms were milder when mothers took supplements.

Probiotics and prebiotics may also be helpful for allergy-proofing. Some trials have found that giving Lactobacillus GG to women with a family history of allergies reduced the risk to their baby of developing eczema. Other studies have found that a combination of probiotics and prebiotics offer similar protection. However, several studies have found that they have no effect. The contradiction may be due to the studies using different strains or doses, but there isn't enough evidence to be sure at the moment.

Probiotics and prebiotics
Probiotics are live micro-organisms, also known as 'friendly bacteria'. They are found naturally in live yogurt, miso and some juices and soya drinks. Prebiotics are food ingredients that aren't digested directly but are consumed by the friendly bacteria in our intestines, helping them to grow at the expense of potentially harmful bacteria. Prebiotics, in the form of fructo-oligosaccharides, are found in bananas, onions and artichokes. Both probiotics and prebiotics can also be taken as supplements.

Seasonal eating and organic food

Eating foods that are in season is often cheaper, tastier, better for the environment and good nutritionally, especially if it means eating more fruit and vegetables. Many people also choose to eat organic food because of environmental concerns and to reduce their exposure to fertiliser and pesticide residues. However, organic food is more expensive and we don't really know if there are any health benefits. Some studies have found particular foods, such as organic carrots, contain higher levels of vitamins or flavonoids, while other studies have found levels are lower, or just the same.

Some people believe that going organic reduces the risks of childhood cancer and early puberty, or that it benefits cognitive development, but there isn't scientific evidence to back this up. The government says that all chemicals used in food, including pesticide sprays and food additives, are tested for safety, and there is no evidence to suggest they are harmful to developing babies. Still, hundreds of new chemicals have been introduced to the food system in the past 60–100 years and nobody knows if long-term effects might be uncovered in years to come. Many women choose to go organic in pregnancy as a precaution to reduce the amount of chemicals they, and therefore their baby, are exposed to. If you're undecided, then bear in mind that the benefits of going organic are debatable, whereas the benefits of eating fruit, vegetables, whole grains, etc., are well established, so these are the areas to focus your attention on.

If you eat organic food, you need to be just as careful about washing fruit and vegetables in order to avoid exposure to harmful bacteria. You should also remember that just because products are organic, it doesn't make them healthy. Organic cola is still sugary water with caffeine and a few additives, and organic chocolate and carrot cake still contain lots of calories. Also, organic food isn't fortified with extra vitamins and minerals, so if you have organic breakfast cereal you could have a lower intake of certain nutrients, such as iron and B vitamins.

Hypospadias and vegetarian diets

Hypospadias is a birth defect in boys in which the opening of the penis isn't at the tip but somewhere further down. What causes this is unknown but it has been linked to genes, medicine and drug use, exposure to environmental pollutants and vegetarianism. In 2000 the results of a study of almost 8,000 babies born in the UK showed hypospadias was five times more common among vegetarians than among non-vegetarians. There was speculation that this could be related to higher intakes of soya among vegetarians, since soya contains a plant oestrogen called genistein. It was also suggested that because vegetarians ate more fruit and vegetables, they were exposed to higher levels of pesticides, which may be to blame. Since 2000, genistein (found in soya) and vinclozolin (a pesticide) have been found to increase the risk of hypospadias and reduce fertility in mice, and a Swedish study among pregnant women has found similar results to the UK study. However, four other studies, including one carried out in south-east England and a very large study from the US, have found no link at all between vegetarianism and hypospadias. These studies found links with workplace exposure to chemicals and hairspray use. On balance, it seems that eating soya beans and products such as tofu and soya milk as part of a balanced diet is fine.

Ice-cream with gherkins and other taste changes

Cravings are quite common in pregnancy, especially during the early stages. They are usually seen as quite a fun part of being pregnant. Whether it's ice-cream with gherkins you're longing for, or something more ordinary like orange juice, when you have it, it'll taste like the best thing ever.

The most common cravings are for fruit, sweet or salty foods and those with a strong flavour, such as pickles. Vegetarians are more likely to crave pickles and savoury or salty foods, whereas cravings for fruit and sweet foods are more common among meat-eaters and fish-eaters. Nobody can explain exactly why cravings occur, but it is thought that changes in hormone levels, particularly oestrogen, are partly responsible. Psychological factors also play a role. In some cultures pregnancy cravings are unheard of. Women sometimes admit that 'cravings' are a good excuse for eating foods they always fancy. It's usually fine to eat the foods you crave, unless they are on the 'avoid list' or are likely to result in you gaining a lot of weight.

There is no evidence that women crave what their body needs, for example craving chalk because they need calcium. However, cravings for things that wouldn't usually be considered a food or drink, such as mud, ice or newspaper, is sometimes a sign of iron deficiency. Cravings such as these are called *pica* and are rare in Western populations: one Danish study found the incidence was just 0.02%. However, they are more common among certain ethnic groups, including African-Americans, and less affluent populations around the world. As several studies have found that pica is associated with low iron levels, if you do find yourself craving something unusual, talk to your doctor or midwife. It may be a good idea to get your iron levels tested if that hasn't yet been done. Also, your doctor or midwife should be able to advise you about the safety or otherwise of eating particular substances.

As well as experiencing cravings, many women find they go off particular foods or drinks during pregnancy. Even the smell of something like wine, which they usually enjoy, can make them feel nauseous. Again, hormonal changes that affect the sense of taste and smell are probably responsible. Aversions to tea, coffee, alcohol, fried or spicy food, and strong flavours and odours are quite normal. For some women, these are the first sign of pregnancy. Aversions to certain items, such as alcohol or coffee, protect a baby from potential harm. However, aversions to healthy foods, such as eggs and vegetables, are not uncommon, particularly when women are suffering from morning sickness. Tastes are likely to return to normal once morning sickness subsides. Part of the problem can be smells from cooking, so it can help if someone else cooks or if you eat more cold foods for a while.

Craving meat?
If you haven't been asked yet, you probably will be. Although some vegetarians crave meat while they're pregnant, the vast majority don't. Research with 40 pregnant lacto-ovo-vegetarians found none of them craved meat. Interestingly, more than 10% of the non-vegetarians in the study went off meat while they were pregnant.

2 Preparing for pregnancy

Whether you are just starting to think about getting pregnant or you are already trying for a baby, this is the ideal time to get your diet and general lifestyle in order. A healthy, balanced diet is important before, as well as during, pregnancy. What you eat now can have an enormous impact on your chances of getting pregnant and of having a healthy baby.

If you make dietary improvements before you become pregnant, they can have a much bigger effect than changes made later. So, rather than burning the candle at both ends while you still have the chance, use this time to prepare your body for a healthy pregnancy. Taking even a few steps in the right direction can help and, as your family grows, you will all reap the health benefits.

You are unlikely to know you are pregnant for about two weeks after you conceive, so it is worth erring on the side of caution when it comes to eating and drinking safely. That means avoiding excess alcohol and caffeine, and thinking more about food hygiene. You might find it helpful to read Chapter 5 to find out which foods and drinks you need to avoid during pregnancy. Then, when you get a positive pregnancy test, you can celebrate without feeling guilty about what you've eaten or drunk over the past few weeks. Also, if you suffer from morning sickness and don't feel like eating, you'll know your body has a good store of nutrients to draw on.

The pre-pregnancy checklist

Do

- Try to reach a healthy weight.
- Take a supplement containing 400µg of folic acid every day. This is important in the very early days after conception, before you know you are pregnant, and will reduce the risks of having a baby with a neural tube defect (see page 134).
- Eat a healthy, balanced diet.
- Be careful about food hygiene (see page 86).
- Exercise to keep fit and relieve stress, but avoid rigorous exercise programmes as these can reduce fertility.
- Talk to your doctor if you have any medical condition, including asthma or epilepsy, or if you are taking any prescription medicines.
- Ask your doctor about the safety of any herbal supplements you are taking. Some that may boost fertility, such as chasteberry, should not be taken during pregnancy.
- Relax and make the most of life. You may get pregnant immediately, but it often takes a while. Stress reduces fertility and there won't be much time for relaxing once you have a new baby to look after.

Don't

- Drink any alcohol or if you do decide to drink, stick to no more than one to two units of alcohol once or twice a week and avoid getting drunk. Drinking more than this reduces fertility and increases the risk of miscarriage. A Swedish study of more than 7,000 women found that drinking more than two units of alcohol per day made getting pregnant more difficult, and even women drinking one or two units per day were more likely to have problems than women drinking less. Moderate alcohol intake is also known to affect development very early in pregnancy. A Danish study found that women drinking more than 10 units of alcohol a week around the time they became pregnant were four times as likely to miscarry.

- Take supplements containing high levels of vitamin A. It is better to stick to supplements specifically for pre-conception.

- Drink too much coffee, tea or other drinks containing caffeine. It is thought that caffeine might affect ovulation. It may also disrupt the smooth rhythmic waves that usually occur in the fallopian tubes to move the egg along to the uterus. It would be sensible to stick to the 200mg caffeine limit for pregnancy (see page 83).

- Smoke, use recreational drugs such as cannabis or take supplements which have not been safety checked for pregnancy, such as evening primrose oil.

What about him?

Creating a healthy baby takes two. There is increasing evidence showing that being a regular drinker and having poor eating habits can lower the quality and quantity of a man's sperm. High intakes of soya have also been linked with reduced sperm quality and, although evidence is patchy, the NHS say that if men with low sperm counts want to reduce their intake of soya products it wouldn't do any harm. A man's lifestyle can even affect birth weight, so it's important that dads-to-be are as healthy as possible. Also, if you both make changes together, such as cutting down on alcohol or fatty foods, it will be much easier. What's more, research has shown time and again that children eat very much like their parents. So if you both get into the habit of eating a healthy balanced diet, there is a much better chance that your baby will too.

The dad-to-be checklist

- Don't drink too much alcohol. Stick within the government's daily limit of no more than 3-4 units daily (equivalent to a pint and a half of 4% beer). Regularly drinking more than this can reduce fertility. The Danish study mentioned above, which found that women drinking more than 10 units a week were more likely to miscarry, also found that if men drank more than this, the pregnancy was more likely to end in miscarriage, even taking into account the woman's alcohol intake.

- Check that you are a healthy weight for your height (see page 17). Men who are overweight or obese (BMI over 25) have been found to have fewer normally moving sperm compared to men who are a healthy weight (BMI 20-24). Sperm DNA fragmentation is also higher in men with a BMI over 25, which reduces the chance of pregnancy. Having a BMI over 29 has been found to have even more significant negative effects on male fertility.

- If your caffeine intake is very high then it may be a good idea to cut down. Some research suggests caffeine makes sperm more lively, which could boost fertility, but other studies suggest high intakes reduce male fertility.

- Eat plenty of zinc-rich foods, including wholegrain cereal products such as bran flakes, wholemeal bread, baked beans and, if you're not a vegetarian, beef, chicken and other meat. Zinc deficiency is linked to reduced testosterone levels and sperm quality.

- Boost your intake of folic acid and antioxidants, particularly vitamin C, by drinking orange juice and eating leafy green vegetables, beans and pulses. These nutrients are important for boosting sperm numbers and making them better swimmers.

- Talk to your doctor if you are taking prescription medication because some, such as certain drugs for hypertension, can affect fertility.

Are walnuts really the secret to healthy sperm?

If you want to be a dad, you need a fistful of walnuts a day, or so news sites and newspapers around the world reported in the summer of 2012. Researchers at the University of California took a group of around 60 healthy men and asked them to eat 75g (about two handfuls) of walnuts every day for three months. They compared these men to a second group who were asked to avoid tree nuts for the same three-month period. At the end of the trial, the walnut eaters showed significant improvements in sperm vitality, motility (movement) and morphology (shape). The benefits were put down to the omega 3 fatty acids found in walnuts, which are thought to be critical for sperm development. Of course, plenty of men become fathers without the aid of walnuts, but it seems walnuts really do affect sperm. A previous study carried out on men attending a fertility clinic found that fish oil supplements, which also contain omega 3 fatty acids, had similar effects on sperm quality.

Assisted conception

If you are trying to get pregnant with IVF or you're having any form of assisted fertility treatment, then it is particularly important that you limit your intake of caffeine and alcohol. NICE (the government's National Institute for Health and Clinical Excellence) has reviewed the research into factors that increase the likelihood of assisted conception treatment being successful. It recommends that couples drink no more than one unit of alcohol per day and avoid having a high caffeine intake. Assisted fertility treatment has also been found to have a much better chance of working if couples are a healthy weight for their height.

Why weight matters

Your weight before you get pregnant can affect your fertility and your baby's health. Being **underweight** can make it more difficult to conceive and increase the risk of miscarriage in the first trimester (three months) of pregnancy. It can also increase the risk of your baby having a very low birth weight or being unwell.

Several studies have shown that being **overweight** is linked to reduced fertility. A study in Denmark found that obese couples were three times more likely to have trouble conceiving than couples of a normal weight. Being overweight also increases the risk of complications during pregnancy, including infections, high blood pressure, preeclampsia, diabetes, and the risk of birth defects, including heart and limb deformities. Another problem is that being overweight makes it more difficult for the midwife to monitor you during pregnancy and labour, and there is a greater chance of problems arising during the birth.

These are of course risks, not certainties, and you are in an ideal position now to do something about your weight and to increase the chances of everything going well.

You can find out if your weight is appropriate for your height by calculating your body mass index (BMI). This can be done either by using an online calculator (**www.nhs.uk/Tools/Pages/Healthyweightcalculator.aspx**) or by following the steps in the box.

Calculating your BMI

By working out your body mass index (BMI) you can see whether you are a healthy weight for your height.

1 Measure your height in metres. To convert from feet and inches to metres, multiply your height in inches by 0.0254. For example, if you are 5ft 2in, this is 62 inches (12 inches to a foot), so the calculation is 62 × 0.0254 = **1.57m**.

2 Take your pre-pregnancy weight in kilograms. To convert from stones and pounds, multiply your weight in pounds by 0.454. For example, if you weigh 10 stones, this is 140 pounds (14 pounds to a stone), so the calculation would be 140 × 0.454 = **63.6kg**.

3 Divide your pre-pregnancy weight by your height squared. In this example:

$$BMI = \frac{63.6}{1.57 \times 1.57} = 25.8$$

For a simpler idea of whether you are the right weight for your height, use the graph given overleaf. First find your height up the side and then your weight along the top or bottom, depending on whether you work in kilograms or in stones and pounds. The NHS uses the following categories:

underweight (BMI less than 18.5), healthy weight (BMI 18.5–25), overweight (BMI 25–30) and obese (BMI over 30). Although a BMI less than 18.5 is used as the cut-off below which general health may suffer, when it comes to getting pregnant, some consider the cut-off should be a BMI of 20, as research has found signs of reduced fertility in women with BMIs below this level.

Height/weight chart

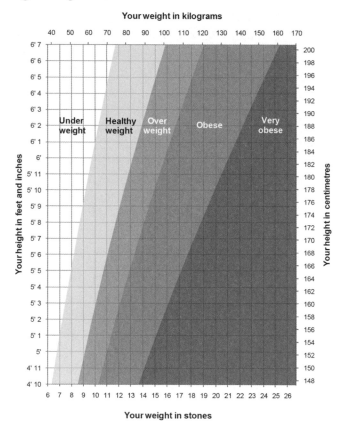

How do you measure up?

Underweight

Many women with a BMI under 20 or even 18.5 don't consider themselves to be underweight. However, having a BMI this low could reduce your chances of getting pregnant and having a healthy baby. The optimal pre-pregnancy BMI is between 20 and 25, based on fertility and healthy pregnancy outcome, but the ideal body weight for individuals varies. Having a BMI of 18 may cause one woman to stop ovulating, while another woman with the same BMI continues to ovulate regularly. Regular periods are sometimes taken as an indicator of normal ovulation, but underweight women may still have regular periods and not actually be ovulating, or not ovulating every month. This is nature's way of ensuring you only become pregnant if your body has enough reserves to support a healthy pregnancy. Becoming pregnant isn't the only issue. One study found that women who became pregnant while they were underweight were 72% more likely to miscarry in the first three months. A certain amount of body fat, around 22%, appears to be needed for women to have normal hormone production, which is necessary for becoming pregnant and staying pregnant.

Even if you feel comfortable with a low BMI, putting on some weight could make all the difference between becoming pregnant or not. In a study of women with unexplained infertility problems attending a clinic in the US, a group of 29 women described as 'fashionably slim' were asked to gain weight. Two of the group were reluctant and decided to drop out, but the others put on weight and 19 of them became pregnant. No other fertility treatment was needed.

To increase your BMI, you should eat regular meals and have larger portions, but still try to have a healthy diet. If you have a small appetite, then choose more energy-dense foods such as full-fat dairy products, nuts, seeds and avocados. You could also use more vegetable oils in cooking or salad dressing. If you find large meals daunting, then don't worry, just eat extra snacks during the day to make up the extra calories you need. If you do a lot of exercise, it might also help to reduce your workouts a bit. If you have a heavy exercise schedule, you may not have an especially low BMI because of the weight of muscle, but your body fat may be below 22%, which could negatively affect fertility.

If you find it difficult to increase your weight, then talk to your GP about getting some help. If you have had an eating disorder in the past, then it's particularly important to ask for support.

Healthy weight

If your BMI is between 18.5 and 25 you are officially in the 'healthy weight' category. However, if your BMI is towards the bottom of the range, below 20, then read the advice for underweight women above. Likewise, women with a BMI at the top of the range should keep an eye on their weight. Otherwise, you don't need to worry and you certainly shouldn't try to lose weight in anticipation of putting it on during pregnancy. Research has shown that women who do this could be putting themselves at increased risk of premature delivery. Instead, you should follow the general advice to ensure you have a healthy diet and get all the nutrients your body needs.

Overweight

If your BMI puts you in the overweight or obese categories, then now is the time to make some changes to your diet and increase your level of physical activity. You've probably tried in the past, but if you need an extra incentive, it may help you to know that losing weight now will affect not only your own health but also the health of your baby.

However, don't try to lose weight too quickly, even if you're keen to get on with the business of baby-making. Strict dieting can deprive your body of the essential nutrients it needs and can actually reduce fertility rather than increase it. Restrictive diets such as the low-carb Atkins diet may seem like a good idea, and some people certainly achieve phenomenal weight loss with this kind of eating. However, research suggests that low-carb diets reduce your chances of becoming pregnant. Likewise, popular diets such as the Dukan diet or the blood group diet aren't balanced, and nobody really knows what affect they might have on fertility or pregnancy.

Still carrying weight from your last pregnancy?
If you've already had a baby and haven't managed to shift the extra weight you put on, then now is the time for action. Mothers who are still carrying the weight gained in their first pregnancy are at increased risk of complications when they become pregnant again. A Swedish study of more than 150,000 women found that even small weight gains could be a problem. Women who rose just one or two BMI units following their first pregnancy (an increase of around 6–12lb) were 20–40% more likely to suffer from high blood pressure or gestational diabetes than those who retained less weight. Gaining more than three BMI units presented further problems, increasing the risk of stillbirth by 60% and the risk of pre-eclampsia by more than 70%.

Crucially, the increased risks didn't just affect women who became overweight or obese following their first pregnancy. They also applied to women who were classified as having a healthy weight for their height, but had gained some weight.

▶

Lingering baby fat is a common problem, even if you have an active toddler or older child to look after. It can be difficult to find time to do much exercise, but going swimming together or getting out to the park regularly is good for everyone. If you're out walking with a pushchair, then you could try upping the pace to help burn calories. Or, if you have an older child, get them on a bike or scooter, then you'll have to run to keep up.

The best strategy is to think longer term and make changes to your eating habits that will help you achieve a slow but steady weight loss. Aim for a pound or two a week (possibly more if you are very overweight, but it's important to do this only with professional advice). A steady weight loss can be achieved by making one or two small changes at a time. Overall you should be aiming to cut down on sugary and fatty foods, and increase your intake of fruit and vegetables, high-fibre foods and water. It's also important to take more exercise.

If you are very overweight, it is worth holding off trying for a baby until after you have lost some of the extra weight. Then you'll have a better chance of everything going well. If you are less overweight, there shouldn't be any problem with you trying for a baby while you lose up to two pounds a week, providing you do it through sensible healthy eating and exercise.

What is a healthy diet?

A healthy diet when you're trying for a baby is basically the same as at any other time. It includes at least five portions of fruit and vegetables a day, plenty of starchy foods such as bread and rice, and some good sources of protein and calcium, such as pulses and dairy foods (see page 32). It's also a good idea to boost your iron intake by having a fortified breakfast cereal, pulses and other iron-rich foods (see page 96). This is because vegetarians tend to have lower iron stores than meat-eaters. If you can build up your iron stores now, you will be less likely to become anaemic during pregnancy.

Omega 3 fatty acids are important for fertility and for foetal brain development, and it can take three months to build up good stores, so now is the time to look at your intake of omega 3 and omega 6 fatty acids. If you're a vegan or don't include much milk in your diet, then it's also important to check that you're having an adequate intake of calcium and vitamin B_{12} (see pages 118 and 110). Vitamin B_{12} is an essential nutrient around the time of conception and works alongside folic acid to help prevent neural tube defects. You should also check that you include some selenium- and iodine-rich foods in your diet. If you already have a baby and he or she is less than a year, or if you've only recently stopped breastfeeding, then healthy eating is especially important, as your stores of key nutrients, including vitamins A and D and omega 3s, may be low.

If you don't usually eat breakfast cereal, you might want to think about starting. A study of nearly 600 pregnant women in Pittsburgh found that those who had eaten cereal regularly around the time of conception (at least three times a week) had significantly higher intakes of folate, iron, zinc, calcium, fibre and vitamins A, C, D and E. These nutrients are all linked to successful placental and foetal development. The researchers suggest that eating cereal is a cheap and easy way to improve nutrient intake in preparation for pregnancy. Many breakfast cereals are highly fortified with these micro-nutrients, but interestingly, women eating any kind of cereal, including unfortified cereals such as muesli, seemed to have higher intakes of these essential vitamins and minerals.

Fertility foods

Adopting a 'fertility diet' could boost your chances of getting pregnant, according to researchers at Harvard University. In a study of more than 17,000 women trying for a baby, they found that those with certain dietary habits and lifestyles were less likely to suffer fertility problems.

The 'fertility diet' they identified was characterised by:

- a high consumption of monounsaturated fats rather than trans fats, e.g. consuming olive oil, nuts and seeds and avoiding processed foods such as cakes and biscuits;
- eating more vegetable protein than animal protein, e.g. avoiding large amounts of meat and eating beans and lentils instead;
- having plenty of low-GI (glycaemic index) carbohydrates rather than high-GI ones, e.g. wholegrain cereals and oats instead of white bread and cakes;
- eating a moderate amount of full-fat dairy produce rather than only low-fat versions of products such as milk and yogurt;
- consuming plenty of vitamins and iron from plant foods and supplements.

Many vegetarians eat these sorts of foods already, but you might want to tweak your diet slightly. The researchers also found that cutting down on alcohol and caffeine was important, as were controlling weight and having a reasonable level of physical activity. When they looked at infertility due to ovulatory disturbances, which is one of the most common fertility problems, they found that women following the diet most closely had a 70% lower risk.

Should you take supplements?

As soon as you stop using contraception you should start taking a folic acid supplement (see page 134). If you are healthy and eating a balanced diet, you shouldn't need to take anything else, although a DHA supplement may be beneficial (see Chapter 8). If you're worried about whether or not you're getting all the nutrients you need then a multivitamin and mineral supplement is a good idea. Make sure you choose a supplement that is specifically for pre-conception and pregnancy. Taking a multivitamin every day has been found to make it more likely that women have regular periods and to increase the chance of getting pregnant. If you take a supplement, think of it as a safeguard for days when you are very busy and can't eat as well as you should: a supplement is not a substitute for healthy eating.

Slugs and snails, or sugar and spice

If you already have a boy or two, and think that a girl would be the icing on the family cake, is there anything you can do to help achieve your ambition? There is certainly plenty of advice out there, but can what you eat really determine the sex of your baby?

It is not guaranteed, but it may be possible to sway the odds slightly. One theory suggests that eating certain foods alters the pH of the vaginal environment, making it more hospitable to X (female) or Y (male) sperm. It seems that X sperm prefer more acidic conditions, while Y sperm fare better in a more alkaline environment. Some believe that the crucial factor is the ratio of sodium and potassium to calcium and magnesium in your diet. If you want a boy, then you need to consume more sodium and potassium, so salty processed foods, plus bananas for potassium. For a girl, it would entail cutting down on these foods and increasing your intake of milk, nuts and pulses.

A recent study involving couples wanting a girl found that following this basic diet principle, along with carefully timed intercourse, really did seem to change the odds. Thirty-two women were prescribed a diet including three glasses of milk a day, plus two portions of yogurt or milk pudding, brown or white rice, salt-free bread or crackers and lots of water to aid calcium absorption. They avoided cheese (because of the high salt content), tea and coffee (high potassium) and also wholemeal bread (potassium plus phytate, which reduces calcium absorption). They also took supplements containing magnesium, calcium and vitamin D and were advised to time intercourse three to four days before ovulation. It was found that 81% of those following the advice conceived a girl. This seems a fairly impressive statistic, but bear in mind that it involved a very small group, the rules were pretty strict, and following this kind of diet long term is not very balanced. Also, we don't know if it was the diet or the timing of intercourse that really had an effect.

Another theory is based on scientists' observations that animals in the wild are more likely to have male offspring if they are fed a richer diet. It has also been found that intentionally increasing the saturated fat intake of mice makes them twice as likely to produce male babies as female babies. In contrast, mice on a low-fat, high-carbohydrate diet are more likely to have female babies. Research looking at the effects of calorie intake and breakfast habits was widely reported when it came out a few years ago. Scientists from the University of Exeter divided women into three groups according to their calorie intake. They found that 56% of those in the high-calorie group had boys, compared to 45%

of those in the low-calorie group. It was suggested that this finding (that eating more calories, like having a higher fat intake, seemed to increase the chances of having a boy) made evolutionary sense, as boy babies are usually bigger. The study also found that 59% of women who ate breakfast cereal daily had a boy, compared to 43% among those who ate cereal less than once a week. The reason for this isn't known, but it could have something to do with higher mineral intakes among cereal eaters.

If you're wondering whether vegetarianism has any effect, it's debatable. A study carried out at Nottingham University found that vegetarians were more likely to have girls. The researchers were actually investigating how the diets of around 6,000 women affected birth weight when they came across this unexpected result. They found that while the national average for Britain is 106 boys born for every 100 girls, the ratio for vegetarian mothers was 85 boys to 100 girls. The researchers couldn't explain the finding and suggested maybe it was related to differing vaginal environments, as the theory above proposes. However, other experts say it may just be a statistical fluke.

On the whole, when it comes to changing your diet in preparation for pregnancy, it is wiser to focus on eating healthily for you and your baby, rather than making adjustments for sex selection. Dietary manipulations, such as eating more salt and saturated fat, or avoiding breakfast, aren't going to give your baby the best start in life, whatever sex they turn out to be. In any case, at best, the diet can only slightly sway the odds of your conceiving a baby that is the 'right sex'. Some experts put the success rate of sex-selection techniques at about 50%, i.e. the same as doing nothing. Alternatively, you could look at methods that don't involve manipulating your diet, such as only having sex at certain stages of your menstrual cycle or changing sexual positions. These are based more firmly on scientific principle and have a better chance of success. To conceive a girl, it may help to have frequent sex after menstruation but to abstain in the two to four days before ovulation. For a boy, avoiding sex in the days before ovulation, and ejaculating deep into the vagina, are advised.

Having trouble conceiving?

If you haven't become pregnant as quickly as you had hoped, try to relax. Of course, this is easier said than done, especially if friends tell you they got pregnant straight away. But the statistics may comfort you: only about 20% of women get pregnant immediately; the other 80% don't. However, around 84% of couples will get pregnant within a year if they are having regular sex without contraception and around 92% within two years.

Before you start worrying about more serious problems, make sure you address simpler issues such as your weight. Both underweight and overweight women increase their chances of conception when they gain or lose weight respectively. An unhealthy lifestyle may not harm some women's chances of getting pregnant. But for others, it can be enough to tip the balance. So, as well as addressing any weight issues you and your partner have, look carefully at every aspect of your diets, including your intake of alcohol and caffeine. Evidence suggests that taking a multivitamin and mineral supplement can also increase the chances of getting pregnant if you've been trying for a while without success. In addition, you might want to look at your intake of vitamin B_6 (see page 107), as a study of Chinese textile workers found that low intakes reduced the women's chances of conception.

Of course, diet is not everything. Don't overlook the obvious issues, such as having regular sex around the time of ovulation. Physical activity is also important – women who are more active before starting fertility treatment, including walking and doing housework, are three times as likely to get pregnant. If you need more advice, the baby charity Tommy's has an excellent guide to pre-pregnancy, which is available free (see Resources, page 186).

If you are still worried and have been trying to get pregnant for more than a year without success (or more than six months if you're over the age of 35), then talk to your GP. This applies to women trying for a second or subsequent baby too. Some mums are surprised they have trouble getting pregnant with baby number two, but 'secondary infertility' appears to be a growing problem.

3 Planning a healthy diet

From conception to birth, a baby needs enormous quantities of nutrients to grow - about 925g of protein, 20-30g of calcium, and a massive 680mg of iron (roughly equivalent to 113 cans of baked beans!). Fortunately, you don't actually need to eat all these extra nutrients, as your body becomes more efficient at extracting them from your food. For example, you are able to absorb four times more iron than usual. These metabolic changes mean your requirements for certain nutrients, including calcium, iron and vitamin B_{12}, are no greater than normal. However, because many young women in the UK currently consume less of these nutrients than is recommended, care is still needed.

The requirements for certain other nutrients, including zinc, thiamine, riboflavin, folate and vitamins A, C and D, are increased for all women during pregnancy.

Although it is essential to get enough of these nutrients overall, you don't need to monitor your intake of each vitamin and mineral every day. Eating a healthy and varied diet, full of wholesome unprocessed foods, will supply most of what you need. If you don't have milk and milk products every day, you also need to find an alternative daily source of calcium and vitamin B_{12}, such as a fortified milk-alternative, and a regular source of iodine. The healthy diet checklist shows the different types of food you should be eating and the main nutrients they supply. Women expecting twins are advised by the NHS to follow the same guidelines as those expecting a single baby.

The healthy diet checklist
A healthy diet for two should include:

- fruit and vegetables to supply vitamins A, C and E, folic acid and iron;
- starchy foods for carbohydrates, B vitamins, iron, zinc and fibre;
- protein foods for essential amino acids, iron, zinc and selenium;
- dairy foods or dairy alternatives for calcium, vitamin B_{12}, iodine and protein;
- iron-rich foods;
- foods supplying folate;
- foods or supplements providing long-chain omega 3s.

Enough calories for two

The total energy cost of pregnancy is estimated to be around 76,000kcal (calories). It sounds like a lot, but don't reach for the biscuit tin just yet. Changes in your metabolism and a reduction in activity levels mean that you don't actually need to increase your calorie intake very much during pregnancy. In fact, for the first six months, women with a healthy pre-pregnancy weight don't need any extra calories at all. Then, during the final three months, when the baby is growing rapidly, they need only 200 extra calories a day.

Appetites vary greatly and some women find they are incredibly hungry at the beginning of pregnancy even though their baby is no bigger than a raisin. This is due to hormonal changes and adjustments the body is already making. Usually this settles down as pregnancy progresses. Energy requirements also vary from person to person according to a variety of factors, including their weight and level of physical activity.

The five food groups

A healthy vegetarian diet for pregnancy is much the same as a healthy diet for anyone. It includes eating foods from the five different food groups in approximately the proportions shown in the 'eatwell plate' overleaf. Using this model can help you plan well-balanced meals. Not every dish has to fit in perfectly, but you should aim for approximately these proportions over a few days. It is a very rough way of ensuring you get most of the nutrients you need and the right balance of macronutrients (protein, carbohydrates and fats). Each food group also tends to provide different micronutrients (vitamins and minerals), so if you don't eat much from one group in particular, you could be missing out some of these. If you think this might be the case, you can find out more about individual vitamins and minerals later in this book (Chapters 6 and 7).

1 Fruit and vegetables

Try to eat at least five portions of a variety of fruit and vegetables every day. This can include fresh, frozen, canned and dried products, as well as juices and smoothies. So, your

The eatwell plate

Use the eatwell plate to help you get the balance right. It shows how much of what you eat should come from each food group.

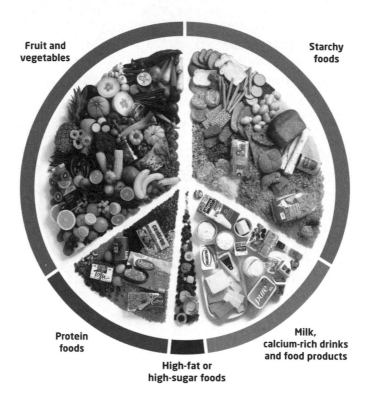

Fruit and vegetables

Starchy foods

Protein foods

Milk, calcium-rich drinks and food products

High-fat or high-sugar foods

Source: Courtesy of the Vegetarian Society, **www.vegsoc.org**

five-a-day could come from a glass of orange juice with breakfast, nuts and raisins mid-morning, salad in a sandwich, and cauliflower and chickpeas in a curry. Fruit juice only counts as one of your five-a-day, no matter how much you have, and the same goes for beans and other pulses. This is because juice contains less fibre than whole fruits, and pulses have fewer micro-nutrients than other vegetables.

Fruit and vegetables don't have to be expensive. Good old carrots provide plenty of health benefits at a fraction of the cost of foods such as blueberries. However, try to eat as wide a variety of differently coloured fruits and vegetables as possible. That way you are more likely to get a full range of different vitamins, minerals and phytochemicals.

Fruit and vegetables are a valuable source of fibre, which is important for digestion and preventing constipation. Adults should consume about 18g of fibre (technically known as non-starch polysaccharides, or NSP) per day. A piece of fruit, such as one apple or orange or a portion of carrots, supplies about 2g. Some vegetables, such as peas, supply more, about 3.5g per portion.

2 Starchy foods

Foods such as breakfast cereals, bread, rice, couscous, potatoes and pasta provide starchy carbohydrates, also known as complex carbohydrates or good carbohydrates. The other kind of carbohydrates is sugars or 'simple carbohydrates', which are found in foods such as white sugar, biscuits and fizzy drinks. Starchy foods should make up about a third of your diet. They are the main source of energy (calories) in our diets and it is good to base each of your meals around one of these foods. It is suggested that about 50% of a person's calories should come from carbohydrates. They contain fewer calories per gram than fat, making carbohydrate-rich foods better than fatty ones for avoiding excess weight gain. The fact that vegetarians tend to eat more carbohydrates and less fat than non-vegetarians partially explains why they are usually slimmer.

It is generally better to eat unrefined starchy foods rather than refined ones. That means foods like wholemeal bread, brown rice and pasta, and wholegrain breakfast cereals (such as bran flakes and muesli), rather than white bread, white rice and pasta, and cornflakes. Wholegrain products provide extra fibre, as you can see in the table below. There are two different types of fibre: insoluble and soluble fibre. Foods such as bran flakes provide insoluble fibre, generally known as roughage, which helps food move through the digestive system, so you don't get constipated. Others, such as oats, provide soluble fibre, which helps to stabilise blood sugar levels.

	Fibre content (g)	Glycaemic load (GL)
Bran flakes (40g bowl)	5	17
Cornflakes (40g bowl)	0.4	41
Granary bread (2 slices)	2.5	18
White bread (2 slices)	1	25
Brown rice (180g)	1.4	19
White rice (180g)	0.3	51

Source: Data taken from various sources including the UK Nutrient Databank © Crown copyright 2012

The impact that a carbohydrate-rich food ('carb') has on blood sugar or blood glucose levels is known as its glycaemic index, or GI. Low-GI foods such as oats and lentils are broken down slowly, so they keep you feeling fuller for longer. As the carbohydrate is released gradually, they produce only a small fluctuation in blood glucose. High-GI foods, by contrast, result in blood sugar levels increasing more rapidly and to a higher level, and then dropping off more steeply. High-GI foods include refined starchy foods such as white bread and also sugary foods like cakes, biscuits and sugary drinks. Less refined foods tend to have a lower GI. For example, the GI is lower for muesli than for bran flakes, which in turn have a lower GI than cornflakes. Likewise, granary bread has a lower GI than wholemeal bread, which has a lower GI than white bread.

To directly compare one food with another, the glycaemic load (GL) is probably more useful as it takes into account the amount of carbohydrate in a typical portion. This makes it easier to assess a food's impact on blood glucose levels. If you want to find the GI or GL of particular foods, there is a wide variety of apps and guidebooks available. Consuming low-GI or low-GL foods as part of a healthy (but not low-calorie) diet has several advantages. Women consuming more low-GI foods are less likely to put on too much weight and there is less risk of their baby being very large. Low-GI diets also reduce the risk of having a baby with a neural tube defect, particularly among overweight women.

As well as helping to stabilise blood sugar levels and providing more fibre, unrefined cereals naturally contain higher levels of certain vitamins and minerals. Wholemeal bread, for example, contains 50% more iron and vitamin B_6 than white bread and more than twice as much potassium and zinc. Unfortunately, high-fibre foods also contain phytate, which binds to certain minerals, including calcium, iron and zinc, and reduces the amount that can be absorbed. Therefore having a very high fibre diet, with foods such as brown rice and lentils, at every single meal isn't necessarily a good thing for maximising mineral absorption. If you eat only unrefined starchy foods, then it might be worth occasionally having white rice or pasta instead. Bran has particularly high phytate levels and is best avoided (see page 151).

Acrylamide

'Could eating burned toast stunt your unborn baby's growth?' asked the *Daily Mail* in 2012. The question arose following a study of acrylamide carried out in 11 maternity units across Europe.

Acrylamide is a chemical that is produced naturally when starchy foods such as potatoes and bread are fried or baked at high temperatures. In the past, it has been linked with cancer, but this study looked at it in relation to pregnancy. The

▶

researchers found that mothers who ate more chips and baked goods had babies with higher levels of acrylamide in their blood. They also found that babies with higher acrylamide levels had lower birth weights and head circumferences. This is the first study to find such an association, and more work is needed to see what is really going on.

The FSA has said there is no need to avoid acrylamide in pregnancy. Even if you wanted to, it would be virtually impossible, as it is found in so many foods. Crisps and chips have particularly high levels, but it's also present at lower levels in bread, breakfast cereals and crisp breads. If you eat a well-balanced diet, you shouldn't have an especially high intake. As an extra precaution you may want to avoid overcooking your chips or toast, and instead have them paler.

3 Protein foods

Protein provides amino acids, the basic building blocks of human tissue. It is needed for the growth of the foetus and placenta and to allow changes in the mother's body that occur during pregnancy. Protein is also required for the production of breast milk. When you are pregnant or breast-feeding, you need about 51g of protein a day. This is just 6g more than before pregnancy. In practice there is usually no need to increase your intake of protein during pregnancy, since the average (non-pregnant) vegetarian woman already consumes more than 51g a day. However, some women have low intakes as their diets consist mainly of vegetables and cereals. It's important to include foods such as chickpeas or lentils whenever you make meals like vegetable curry or chilli to boost the protein content. Women sometimes consider taking a protein supplement, but these are unnecessary. It is much better to eat real foods; then you'll also be getting a whole range of other vital nutrients too.

Lacto-ovo-vegetarians tend to get much of their protein from milk and milk products, but it's important to eat a variety of different protein-rich foods, such as beans and lentils, as these provide iron, B vitamins and fibre too. Relying too heavily on cheese means having a high intake of salt and saturated fat. Plant sources of protein are sometimes described as being of low biological value because they contain fewer essential amino acids than proteins from animal sources. However, you can get all the amino acids you need by eating a variety of different cereals, peas, beans, lentils, seeds and nuts. If you don't usually do this, it is a good idea to start trying to include a source of protein in every meal.

	Grams of protein per 100g	Protein per portion
Baked beans	5	10g per half-tin
Chickpeas	7	8g per half-tin
Kidney beans	7	8g per half-tin
Lentils	7.5	9g in 3 tablespoons
Tofu	8	8g per quarter-pack
Vegetarian sausages	15	15g in two sausages
Nut cutlet	5	5g per cutlet
Quorn mince or pieces	14	11g per quarter-pack
Brazil nuts, hazelnuts, pine nuts, walnuts	14	4.5g per 30g handful
Peanuts	25	7.5g per 30g handful
Muesli	10	5g per 50g bowl
Bread	9	8g in two slices
Milk	3.5	10g per half-pint/ 300ml
Yogurt	5	7g per small pot
Eggs	12.5	14.0g in two eggs

Source: Data taken from various sources including the UK Nutrient Databank © Crown copyright 2012

4 Milk, calcium-rich drinks and food products

Cow's milk and dairy foods such as cheese and yogurt provide protein, calcium, iodine and vitamins A and B_{12}. Full-fat dairy foods also contain saturated fat and can be quite high in calories. It is healthier to choose semi-skimmed, 1% fat, or skimmed milk, as well as reduced-fat cheeses and low-fat yogurts. However, be careful with flavoured yogurts that are described as 'diet' or fat-free, as these can have lots of added sugar.

If you avoid dairy products, it's important to have other foods that supply the same nutrients. A milk-alternative made from soya will provide almost as much protein as cow's milk and, if it's fortified, you'll get calcium, vitamin D and vitamin B_{12} as well. You can also get calcium and vitamin B_{12} from other foods (see Chapter 7). Getting enough iodine on a vegan diet can be more difficult as it is found in only a small number of foods, but some seaweeds are very iodine-rich (see page 121).

5 High-fat or high-sugar foods

Foods such as margarine, cooking oils, cakes, crisps and fizzy drinks are all included in this group.

Fat gets a bad press, but some fatty acids (the building blocks for fat) are essential for good health. There are three main types of fatty acid, which are found in varying amounts in foods:

- Saturated - the type found in meat and dairy products such as cheese. These are not essential, and a high intake increases the risk of heart disease.

- Monounsaturated - found in olive oil and rapeseed oil. These are considered healthy but are also not essential to health.

- Polyunsaturated – some polyunsaturated fatty acids (PUFAs) are known as 'essential fatty acids'. They can't be produced by the body and must be supplied by the diet. There is more information about the omega 3 and omega 6 PUFAs later in this book (Chapter 8).

As well as providing essential fatty acids, fat is needed for the absorption of the fat-soluble vitamins A, D, E and K. It is estimated that about 30g of fat is needed each day. However, fat shouldn't make up more than 35% of your calorie intake.

Trans fats
Trans fats have a similar effect on health as saturated fats – they raise blood cholesterol levels and increase the risk of heart disease. Small amounts of trans fats are found naturally in meat and dairy foods. They are also found in hydrogenated vegetable oil, which is sometimes used for frying and in processed foods such as cakes, biscuits and pastries, as a cheap way of increasing their shelf-life. You shouldn't have more than 5g of trans fats per day.

Some sources of fat are obvious, such as cooking oils, but many foods like pastry, cheese, flapjacks and peanut butter have hidden fats. The fat in nuts and seeds is 'good fat', but eating too much still means having more calories than are needed.

High-sugar foods, such as cakes, sweets and fizzy drinks, are also in this group. They contain refined sugar and provide calories but few or no useful nutrients. Another problem is that these foods have a high GI, so they produce a spike in your blood sugar levels and affect the amount of sugar your baby is exposed to. If your blood glucose is too high then

	Grams of fat per 100g	Fat per portion
Cooking oil (e.g. olive, sunflower)	99.9	5g per teaspoon
Butter	82	4g per teaspoon
Margarine	82	4g per teaspoon
Cheddar	34	10g per 30g portion
Reduced-fat Cheddar	22	7g per 30g portion
Peanut butter	51	5g per teaspoon
Pizza	8-12	14-17g per half pizza
Chocolate	25-40	12-20g per 50g bar
Flapjack	20-27	8-10g per flapjack
Carrot cake	22	17g per 75g slice
Crisps	30-32	10g per 30g bag

Source: Data taken from various sources including the UK Nutrient Databank © Crown copyright 2012

your baby will grow too fast and have an excess amount of body fat.

Sugars are also found in fruit and milk, but these foods are not included in this food group. They are considered healthy because the sugar in them is produced naturally and they also contain other nutrients, including vitamin C and calcium. They also have a lower GI, so have less impact on your blood sugar levels. With fruit, this is because the sugar is more difficult to digest than it is in products like biscuits, so it leads to a slower rise in blood glucose levels. For milk and milk products, the sugar is accompanied by protein, which has a similar effect. Fruit juice, however, has a higher GI and contains less fibre than fruit, so it is best to have no more than one glass of juice per day.

Ten healthy snacks

Snacks are particularly important during pregnancy, whether you're suffering from morning sickness or heartburn, or just feeling hungrier than usual. Snacks such as these will boost your nutrient intake and keep you going until your next meal:

1 Dairy or soya yogurt sprinkled with seeds.
2 A piece of fresh fruit.
3 A handful of dried fruit and nuts.
4 A bowl of cereal, preferably a high-fibre one with added vitamins and iron.
5 Oatcakes with low-fat cheese or vegan cheese.
6 Lentil and vegetable soup.
7 Wholemeal toast with yeast extract, cream cheese or mashed banana.
8 Houmous and vegetable sticks.
9 A milkshake or soyashake made with banana, strawberries, mango or peach.
10 A bowl of muesli with fruit and yogurt.

Fluids

During pregnancy you need to drink around eight glasses or mugs of fluid a day, and more if it's hot or you're exercising. Your fluid intake can include water, tea, coffee, juice or milk, although caffeine intake should be limited (see page 83) as should fruit juice and fizzy drinks (see above). Plain water is an obvious alternative, but you could also try decaffeinated tea or coffee or fruit teas.

Sometimes pregnant women are tempted to restrict their fluid intake in order to avoid going to the toilet so often, or they think it might ease problems with water retention.

However, needing to wee frequently is caused by hormonal changes in early pregnancy, so not drinking isn't likely to help. Also, restricting fluid intake can actually make water retention worse. If you have swollen ankles and wrists, drinking more might actually improve matters. Drinking plenty will also help you avoid constipation. Increasing the amount of fibre you eat without having a good fluid intake can make constipation worse, as dietary fibre needs to absorb water to help it move through the intestines. A good fluid intake will also dilute your urine, which will help to protect you from urinary tract infections.

Choosing fortified foods

We generally think the healthiest foods are unprocessed and just as nature intended. On the whole this is true: highly processed diets certainly contribute to many of today's health problems. However, eating a few fortified foods alongside unprocessed ones can change a deficient diet into a very healthy one. This applies to everyone to some extent, but for vegans fortified foods are particularly important to ensure a good intake of calcium, and vitamins D and B_{12}. It is good to look out for fortified foods generally, for example if you're buying a vegeburger mix, but it's particularly important to find fortified foods that you like and can eat every day, such as breakfast cereals and milk-alternatives. Most nutrients are better absorbed if in small amounts, so getting them from different foods throughout the day is better than having them all at once in a supplement pill.

There are so many cereals available that it can be tricky to find a healthy one. Wholegrain products that are low in salt and sugar are best, and choosing one with added iron can make a real difference to your overall iron intake. The average adult (including meat-eaters) gets 44% of their iron from cereals and cereal products. For vegans and lacto-ovo-vegetarians who don't have much dairy, it's good to look for one that is also fortified with vitamins B_{12} and D. Some 'healthy' cereals, such as bran flakes, have added vitamins and iron, but others, like muesli and Shredded Wheat, don't. Organic cereals never have these nutrients added, as this is against the UK's organic certification rules, though it is allowed in the US. Often 'free from' products don't have them added either, for example gluten-free cereals. Some budget brands, such as supermarkets' own 'basics' ranges, have one nutrient added but not another, while some cheaper cereals are fortified better than expensive brands. There doesn't seem to be any pattern, so you just have to read the labels. If you don't want to eat products fortified with vitamin D_3 (see page 114), then it's still a good idea to find one with added iron and vitamin B_{12}.

If you're looking for a milk-alternative then try to find one with added calcium and vitamins B_{12} and D. Most soya milks are fortified with these, but organic ones aren't. Likewise rice and oat milks tend to have all three micro-nutrients added, but coconut milk may have calcium but not vitamins B_{12} or D. Another good source of vitamin B_{12} is yeast extract, although not all brands are fortified (see page 109). Other fortified foods to look out for are orange juice with added calcium, and many soya products.

Planning meals

If you're not a very adventurous cook, now is a good time to start experimenting with different ingredients. By eating a variety of pulses, nuts, starchy foods and vegetables, you're more likely to get all the nutrients you need. Making your own meals is usually healthier and cheaper and needn't take any longer than cooking convenience foods. If you usually live on pasta, baked potatoes and cheese, you can find inspiration by getting a new cook book or looking online for recipes. The Vegetarian Society and the Vegan Society websites both include great recipes and ideas for easy meals. When you have a bit more time, you can make meals in bulk, such as dahl, chickpea curry, quorn chilli or pasta sauce with lentils; then you can still have a healthy meal when you're in a hurry.

The one-week meal plans below show how you can get all the nutrients you need from meals and snacks if you are a lacto-ovo-vegetarian or a vegan. They aren't meant to be carefully followed, but they give you an idea of what a healthy balanced diet looks like. Each of the weekly menu plans meets the recommendations for the essential minerals: calcium, copper, iodine, magnesium, phosphorus, potassium and selenium; as well as the important vitamins: folate, niacin, riboflavin, thiamine, and vitamins A, B_6, B_{12} and C.

The menu plans don't mention fluids, though these are also important and it is assumed drinks would be included throughout the day. Also, like most diets, they do not provide enough vitamin D, and although you should get some vitamin D from going out in the sun, you should also take a supplement in order to meet the recommended intake.

Vegan – one-week menu plan

MONDAY

Breakfast	Wholemeal toast with almond butter and a glass of orange juice*
Lunch	Lentil soup, granary roll with margarine* and an apple
Dinner	Stir-fried tofu, broccoli and red pepper (with Kombu) and white rice

Snacks	Banana and oat milk* shake, slice of toast with margarine* and Marmite*

TUESDAY

Breakfast	Grapefruit, bran flakes* and oat milk*
Lunch	Baked beans on granary toast with margarine*, couple of satsumas
Dinner	Baked potato with margarine*, veggy sausages with gravy, peas and carrots
Snacks	Flapjack, handful of brazil nuts and raisins

WEDNESDAY

Breakfast	Hot oat cereal* made with soya milk*, sprinkled with chopped nuts and seeds
Lunch	Lentil cutlet and salad in pitta bread, milkshake made with oat milk*
Dinner	Chickpea biryani with chapatti and mango chutney, fruit salad
Snacks	Carrot cake (homemade with margarine*), handful of dried apricots

THURSDAY

Breakfast	Fruit and fibre* with oat milk*, glass of orange juice*
Lunch	Wholemeal pitta with houmous and carrot sticks, slice of melon
Dinner	Pasta with lentil and tomato sauce, apple pie with vegan cream*
Snacks	Handful of brazil nuts, oaty biscuits

FRIDAY

Breakfast	Nutty muesli, hemp milk* and sliced strawberries
Lunch	Wrap with houmous, falafel, avocado, lettuce and tomato
Dinner	Mixed bean and vegetable chilli (with kombu and Marmite*) with rice, pear
Snacks	Handful of mixed dried fruit and nuts, slice of cake (homemade with margarine*)

SATURDAY
Breakfast   Bran flakes* with hemp milk* and sliced banana
Lunch   French bread with vegan cheese, pickle and tomato,
             glass of orange juice*
Dinner   Beanburger, chips and ketchup, corn-on-the-cob with
             margarine* and salad, raspberries and soya yogurt*
Snacks   Breadsticks with lentil dip, dried prunes

SUNDAY
Breakfast   Granary toast with margarine* and Marmite*, mixed
             berries with soya yogurt* and a sprinkling of mixed seeds
Lunch   Vegetable soup and wholemeal roll with margarine*, slice of
             vegan chocolate cake
Dinner   Shepherd's pie made with soya mince, rhubarb crumble
             and custard made with oat milk*
Snacks   Crumpets with peanut butter and jam, an apple

*These foods and drinks are fortified and this makes all the difference between reaching the recommended amount for certain nutrients or not, particularly for vitamin B_{12} and calcium. You'll also notice the odd sprinkling of kombu for iodine and some brazil nuts for selenium – without these, this menu plan would be deficient in these two minerals.

Lacto-ovo-vegetarian – one-week menu plan

MONDAY
Breakfast   Bran flakes with milk and chopped banana
Lunch   Cheese and tomato toasted sandwich with
             wholemeal bread, an orange
Dinner   Chickpea curry with basmati rice, yogurt and mango
             chutney; a crème caramel
Snacks   Apricot flapjack, handful of brazil nuts

TUESDAY
Breakfast   Porridge topped with honey and chopped nuts and seeds

Lunch	Wholemeal pitta bread filled with houmous, avocado and red pepper salad and a glass of orange juice
Dinner	Stir fried tofu, broccoli, carrot and baby corn with egg noodles
Snacks	Date and walnut cookie, a pear

WEDNESDAY

Breakfast	Wholemeal toast with peanut butter and mashed banana
Lunch	Lentil soup, granary roll with margarine; slice of banana bread
Dinner	Vegetable lasagne, salad and a fruit yogurt
Snacks	Homemade milkshake (strawberries and milk), a cereal bar

THURSDAY

Breakfast	Weetabix-type-cereal with chopped banana and almonds
Lunch	Baked potato with baked beans and a spoonful of grated cheese; a peach
Dinner	Vegetarian sausages and gravy, oven chips, peas and carrots
Snacks	Wholemeal toast with scraping of margarine and Marmite, small fruit smoothie

FRIDAY

Breakfast	Nutty muesli with milk
Lunch	Egg mayonnaise sandwich with wholemeal bread, small packet of crisps and pot of fruit salad
Dinner	Vegetable and bean chilli, basmati rice; mixed berries with yogurt and honey
Snacks	Dried prunes, chocolate biscuit

SATURDAY

Breakfast	Bran flakes with milk, glass of orange juice
Lunch	Wrap with falafel, lettuce, tomato and yogurt dressing
Dinner	Vegetable pizza with mixed salad, ice-cream
Snacks	Mixed nuts and raisins, a fruit bun

SUNDAY

Breakfast	Scrambled eggs, toast, mushrooms and tinned tomato
Lunch	Quorn fillet, new potatoes, broccoli and cauliflower cheese and carrots; apple crumble and custard
Dinner	Roast vegetable soup, rye bread with cream cheese and grapes
Snacks	Chocolate-coated brazil nuts

4 A healthy weight gain for pregnancy

The amount of weight women gain during pregnancy varies enormously. The extra weight isn't just the baby; it is also the placenta, amniotic fluid, increased blood volume and extra tissue in the breasts and uterus. It is also natural to lay down extra fat so that you have energy stores for breast-feeding. Some women have fluid retention during pregnancy, which contributes further to weight gain.

The general advice is that if you eat according to your appetite then you should gain a healthy amount of weight. Unfortunately many women these days aren't used to eating in response to hunger and fullness, especially those who have been yo-yo dieters or particularly weight-conscious in the past. Some women become quite anxious about putting on weight and may try to restrict their weight gain. Others take the opposite view and see pregnancy as a time to relax their usual rules about avoiding fattening foods and instead eat whatever they fancy. Neither approach is good, as gaining too little or too much weight can cause problems.

How much weight should you gain?

The amount of weight you should gain during pregnancy depends on your weight before you became pregnant. Women who are overweight need to gain much less than those who are underweight to produce a healthy baby.

You can find out if you were in the 'underweight', 'healthy weight' or 'overweight' category before pregnancy using pages 17 and 18, and then using the guidelines in the table here see roughly how much weight you should gain during pregnancy. The recommendations come from the Institute of Medicine in the USA and they have been calculated using data from thousands of women. Weight gains within the recommended ranges are associated with the lowest risk of complications during pregnancy and labour (including the need for a caesarean) and the best chances of having a healthy baby whose weight is within the normal healthy range. Women with weight gains within the recommended range are also less likely to have lots of weight to lose after having their baby, and their baby is less likely to become overweight or obese.

BMI before pregnancy	Recommended weight gain
Underweight, less than 18.5	12.5–18kg (2st to 2st 12lb)
Healthy weight, 18.5–25	11.5–16kg (1st 11lb to 2st 7lb)
Overweight, 25–30	7–11.5kg (1st 1lb to 1st 11lb)
Obese, more than 30	5–9kg (11lb to 1st 6lb)

Source: Data from Institute of Medicine (2009) *Weight Gain During Pregnancy: Re-examining the Guidelines*. National Academies Press, Washington, DC.

The weight gain ranges in the table look fairly broad and at first glance you may think that they look easily achievable.

Weight gain chart

Monitor your weight by marking with an X throughout your pregnancy.

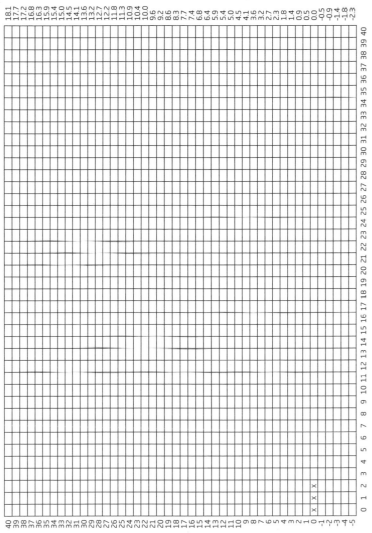

Weight gain (kg)

Weight gain (pounds)

Week of pregnancy

However, the majority of women in the UK and the USA gain either too much or too little weight. Weighing yourself regularly during pregnancy may help you stay on track. You can use the graph on the previous page to keep a record of your weight gain and see how it compares to the recommendations.

Some women find it easier if, rather than thinking about the whole nine months, they take their pregnancy in stages. You might have read that you don't need to gain any weight during the first trimester (three months) of pregnancy, but in reality most women put on between 0.5 and 2.5kg (1 to 6lb). During the second and third trimesters, women in the 'underweight' or 'normal weight' category should gain about 0.5kg (1lb) per week and 'overweight' or 'obese' women should gain about 0.25kg (0.5lb) each week.

If you're concerned about gaining too much or too little weight, it is important to talk to your GP or midwife about your worries. Remember that there is not an exact amount of weight that you should be putting on, and women with a wide range of weight gains have good pregnancies and healthy babies. Your GP or midwife will be able to tell you whether or not you need to be doing anything about your weight gain, not only based on the number on the scales, but also taking into account how your baby appears to be growing and your general health.

Making sure you gain enough weight

There is a very strong association between weight gain during pregnancy and birth weight. The more weight you put on, the bigger your baby is likely to be. Your weight before pregnancy is also important, and if you start off lighter then you need to gain more weight to have a baby that's a healthy weight. Some women feel that a small baby isn't such a problem, and that it should make labour easier anyway. However, low-birth-weight babies are more likely to have problems at birth and in later life (see page 3).

If you've been particularly weight conscious in the past or have had an eating disorder, such as anorexia nervosa or bulimia nervosa, you may feel particularly anxious about gaining weight during pregnancy. If this is the case it's good to talk to your GP or midwife about your concerns. They may offer extra appointments to monitor your baby's growth and they should be able to help you deal with your concerns or refer you to someone who can.

Vegetarians, and vegans in particular, tend to weigh less than meat-eaters. Healthy diets, which are low in fat, high in fibre and contain lots of fruit and vegetables, can have a low energy density, which means you don't get a lot of calories per mouthful. This is generally considered a benefit, but if you're finding it difficult to eat enough calories then you could try some of the following:

- Include more energy-dense foods in your meals, such as cheese, nut butters, beans and lentils.
- Cook with a little more oil, such as olive oil or rapeseed oil.
- If you have a salad, add some avocado, a handful of seeds and some salad dressing.
- Have a mid-morning and mid-afternoon snack such as dried fruit and nuts, flapjack, oatcakes and cheese.
- Eat breakfast every day.
- Have a milky drink before bed, such as a fortified malt drink like Ovaltine, or a chocolaty soya milk such as Vitasoy or Alpro chocolate shake. Or make your own milkshake-type drink with a fortified milk such as soya, rice, almond, coconut or hemp milk, blended with a banana and some nut butter.

Making sure you don't gain too much weight

Several studies have found that vegetarian women are less likely than others to put on too much weight during pregnancy, but weight is an issue for an increasing number of women.

Gaining more weight than recommended increases your risk of complications during pregnancy, including gestational diabetes, high blood pressure and pre-eclampsia. It also increases the chances of your having a very large baby, which can increase the risks during delivery, including the need for a caesarean. In addition, it increases your own risks of being obese in the future, which in turn means that you are more likely to develop heart disease, diabetes and cancer.

Some women take the attitude that they won't worry about their weight for now, they'll just eat what they like and enjoy being pregnant, then they'll lose the weight afterwards. Unfortunately, losing weight after pregnancy isn't as easy as many celebrities would have you believe. A Swedish study found that women who gained more than 16kg (2.5 stone) during pregnancy were on average 5.5kg (12lb) heavier a year after their baby was born. For some women, the effects can still be seen many years after having a baby. A study of more than 2,000 women in the UK found that those gaining more weight than recommended were three times more likely to be overweight 16 years later. Similar results were found in a group of Australian women 21 years after they had had their babies.

The O word

Nobody likes to be described as obese, but if your BMI is over 30 you are likely to hear doctors and midwives using the word. It's not meant to be judgemental or offensive;

it's a clinical word used to make sure you get the care you need during pregnancy. This might mean extra monitoring or antenatal appointments, or special facilities may be needed during the birth of your baby.

In the spring of 2012 many newspapers reported that 'dieting in pregnancy was good for you' and that expectant mothers were being 'urged to go on a diet'. The stories were based on a paper that appeared in the *British Medical Journal* (BMJ), which found that following a healthy diet plan (not a weight-loss diet) helped women not to put on too much weight during pregnancy. It was actually an analysis of the results of more than 30 different trials that had looked at different ways of managing weight gain in pregnancy. It was found that the best way to avoid putting on too much weight was to follow healthy eating advice, including eating low-fat foods and those with a low glycaemic index (GI) (see page 36). Exercise helped some women keep their weight under control, but exercise alone, without healthy eating, wasn't generally very effective. The really important finding was that when women followed advice regarding diet and exercise, neither their baby's birth weight nor health was affected, which is something many women worry may happen if they don't eat what their body seems to want. In fact, the risk of some complications, including pre-eclampsia, was reduced.

So it seems that taking steps to control weight gain can benefit both you and your baby. But it is important to take a sensible approach. We know that women who are overweight are more likely to have conditions such as high blood pressure, diabetes and problems during labour, but going on a strict diet now won't benefit you or your baby. Dieting to lose weight during pregnancy is associated with an increased risk of neural tube defects and other complications. If you weigh more than about 100kg or 16 stone, your GP or midwife may feel that a calorie-controlled diet is appropriate, with careful monitoring.

Although now is not the time for dieting, it is good to develop healthier eating habits. The important thing is to try to make a conscious effort every day to eat as healthily as possible and increase the amount of time you spend walking or taking gentle exercise. These healthier habits will stand you in good stead for when your baby is born and then you can think seriously about achieving a healthy weight for the long term. You can still have the occasional treat, but factor these in to the overall plan. For example, if you have a few chocolate biscuits or other treats one afternoon, don't think 'healthy eating is ruined for today'. Instead try to eat as healthily as possible later on. If you find you're constantly tempted by high-fat and high-sugar foods, such as crisps or chocolate, then make sure you always have healthier options available – see 'Ten healthy snacks' (page 43). Also try eating more low-GI foods to stabilise your blood sugar levels and keep you feeling fuller for longer. The aim of healthy eating is to get the right combination of nutrients while getting enough, but not too many, calories. This is something vegetarians are often better at than meat-eaters, but it's not always the case.

One thing that recent studies have shown is that monitoring your weight gain and having a plan really helps. As well as using the graph (page 53) you can set yourself small targets, such as taking fruit to work instead of having biscuits. Or, cut down from two sugars in tea to just one and a half, then in a couple of weeks you could cut down to one sugar. Set goals that you feel are achievable and that you think you can stick to in the long term. Also, don't let other people spoil your good intentions by telling you that you need an extra roast potato or biscuit because you're eating for two.

Low-carb eating

Low-carb diets, such as the Atkins diet, could be dangerous during pregnancy. They can lead to your baby laying down extra fat, and the proportion of the diet made up of protein inevitably increases, which is also undesirable. Animal studies show protein-rich diets increase the risk of miscarriage and genetic abnormalities. Studies carried out in Scotland have also shown that a high protein intake during pregnancy makes babies more susceptible to raised blood pressure, insulin sensitivity and heart disease in later life. Low-carb eating for vegetarians is also likely to mean a very high intake of eggs, tofu or commercially prepared high-protein foods or shakes. The effects of these are unknown but they are unlikely to be beneficial.

How to gain a healthy amount of weight

NICE have identified the following strategies as really helping women to achieve a healthy weight gain:

- eat breakfast;
- watch your portion sizes (don't eat for two);
- base meals around starchy foods such as potatoes and rice;
- eat fibre-rich foods, such as oats, wholegrain products and vegetables;
- make sure you get your five-a-day;
- eat a low-fat diet;
- avoid high-fat and high-sugar foods, such as fried food, fast food, fizzy drinks and cakes.

Keeping active

As well as thinking about what you eat, it's important to stay active to avoid putting on too much weight. Getting out and keeping physically active is also essential for your general sense of well-being. This means avoiding spending long periods sitting and watching TV or using the computer, and instead making walking part of your daily life. Taking some exercise will help you feel healthier and more relaxed, and as a bonus you're likely to sleep better. If you are fit, you are also likely to have more stamina for labour and an easier birth. In addition, it'll help you recover more easily after the birth and make you feel more energetic and better able to look after your baby.

The NHS recommends at least 30 minutes of moderate exercise per day during pregnancy. This can include swimming or brisk walking. If you took little or no exercise before pregnancy, it is best to start with just 15 minutes per day and build up gradually. Most leisure centres hold classes that are specifically for pregnant women, such as prenatal aqua aerobics, or you could find out if there are antenatal yoga classes nearby. These are also a good way to meet other mums-to-be. If you feel you really don't have time to go to a class, then any exercise, even a 10-minute walk around the block, is better than nothing.

Twins and more!

If you are expecting twins, triplets or even more babies, you are likely to gain more weight than a woman expecting just one baby. This is due to the weight of an extra baby but also to an extra placenta and more amniotic fluid. You are likely to feel particularly hungry in early pregnancy and gain more weight in the first few months.

The amount of weight that women expecting twins should gain during pregnancy has been calculated by the Institute of Medicine (IOM) in the USA. The recommendations are based on evidence of weight gains associated with the healthiest outcomes for mums and their babies. The IOM describes these guidelines as 'provisional' as there is not as much data available for twin pregnancies. However, since there are no other recommendations available, you might find them useful. If you were underweight before you became pregnant, you might notice that there is no recommendation for you in the table here. This is because there was simply not enough data available for the IOM to base one on. However, you should aim to gain slightly more than is recommended for 'healthy weight' women.

BMI before pregnancy	Recommended weight gain
Healthy weight, 18.5-25	17-25kg (2st 9lb to 3st 12lb)
Overweight, 25-30	14-23kg (2st 3lb to 3st 8lb)
Obese, more than 30	11-19kg (1st 11lb to 3st)

Source: Data from Institute of Medicine (2009) *Weight Gain During Pregnancy: Re-examining the Guidelines.* National Academies Press, Washington, DC.

There are no official guidelines regarding additional energy and calorie requirements for multiple pregnancies. However, extra calories are needed, and these should come from nutrient-rich foods rather than extra sugary or fatty foods. The additional foods also need to supply extra vitamins and minerals, including iron and vitamin A, which are more likely to be lacking in multiple pregnancies.

5 Foods and drinks to avoid and those you don't need to

When you are pregnant you should avoid certain foods and drinks, and cut down on others. Some, such as raw eggs, can cause food poisoning, and others, like coffee, could be toxic to your baby if you have too much.

If you flick through this chapter, you might be shocked at the number of pages of foods that you now can't eat. However, it is quite likely that you don't eat half of them anyway. Some women feel that the government advice is too cautious and that there really isn't much risk of their getting food poisoning. It's true the chances of a woman getting any form of food poisoning are very small, and even smaller for those who don't eat meat, poultry or seafood, as these are the most common culprits. However, during pregnancy you are more likely than normal to get sick from something you eat. It is estimated that you are about 20 times more likely than usual to get listeriosis. This is because your immune system undergoes several changes to stop your body rejecting your growing baby.

There are about 1.7 million cases of food poisoning in England and Wales each year, according to the Health

Protection Agency (HPA). The HPA estimates that toxoplasmosis affects two in every 1,000 pregnant women in the UK, and that there are 20 to 30 cases of listeriosis among pregnant women every year. The numbers are small, but since infection could result in miscarriage or stillbirth, it is understandable that women are advised to avoid particular foods. Ultimately it is up to the individual to assess whether any risk is worth taking.

If you eat something and later realise it is on the 'avoid' list, try to keep things in perspective. The chances of getting food poisoning on any single occasion are extremely small. Even if you do feel unwell, it may just be a coincidence. However, if you're feeling sick it is best to see your doctor, as they can assess whether you might have listeria or any other form of food poisoning. They can also arrange testing and treatment in the unlikely event that it's needed.

Who decides what's safe?
In the UK the Food Standards Agency (FSA) is responsible for food safety and food hygiene. It bases its advice for pregnant women on the most up-to-date evidence from research studies and surveys. Eating food, like crossing the road or just about any other activity, carries some risk. Any food could be potentially dangerous. In recent years there have been cases of salmonella in products as diverse as chocolate and watermelons. The FSA knows that listeria could be present in any ready-to-eat food, including dips, sandwiches and salads, but advising people to avoid such a large range of foods wouldn't be practical or healthy. Instead it considers which foods have most often been linked to food poisoning, and identifies those with the highest risk. Pregnant women are advised to avoid a particular food only if it has consistently been found to pose a risk to health, and the

consequences of eating it are thought to be significant. By taking into account all the evidence, it is possible to balance the health benefits against the potential risk for foods such as eggs, blue cheese or pâté.

Before blaming the 'Food Police' for banning everything tasty, it is worth trying to put things in perspective. There's actually very little that's completely off limits when you're pregnant. The foods that make up the bulk of our everyday diets, such as bread, cereals and different types of milk, can still be enjoyed guilt-free, as can occasional treats such as cookies and chips. As a vegetarian you don't need to worry about advice regarding foods such as liver and oysters, and most of us don't usually eat foods such as homemade mayonnaise anyway. However, there are bound to be some changes that you should make. For example, if your favourite cheese is Brie, you'll need to have it hot or find an alternative, such as a mature Cheddar; and if you do usually start the day with a pot of coffee, it would be wise to switch to decaf.

Checklist of foods to avoid

During pregnancy these foods pose a risk to you or your baby:

- Soft mould-ripened cheeses, including blue-veined varieties (see page 68).
- Raw or partially cooked eggs (see page 71).
- Unpasteurised milk and milk products.
- Pâté (listeria risk).

- Unwashed fruit and vegetables.
- Raw bean sprouts.
- Alcohol.
- Caffeine (avoid having more than 200mg per day).

Some women worry about having food additives, but the FSA considers all additives used in the UK to be safe for consumption during pregnancy and while breastfeeding. Having an additive-laden diet isn't ideal, however: there are concerns that consuming a range of additives could have a 'cocktail effect', and if you're consuming lots of additives then you're eating processed foods which are probably high in sugar, salt and fat and low in micro-nutrients. A diet made up primarily of unprocessed foods is inevitably healthier.

Milk and milk products

While you are pregnant, it is best to avoid drinking raw or unpasteurised milk (including goats' or sheep's milk) or using it in cooking. Unpasteurised milk may contain listeria and other bacteria, such as *E. coli* and brucella, which can cause food poisoning.

It is safe to drink milk that is pasteurised or heat-treated to kill harmful bacteria, including UHT milk, powdered milk, evaporated milk and condensed milk. Milk products made from pasteurised milk are also fine, including butter, cream, soured cream, clotted cream, crème fraiche, fromage frais, cottage cheese and yogurt.

Raw or unpasteurised milk and milk products are not widely available, but they may be sold on the Internet or at farm shops or farmers' markets.

Cheese

Some cheeses should not be eaten during pregnancy because of the risk of listeria. The general rule is that soft mould-ripened cheeses (e.g. Brie) and soft blue cheeses (e.g. Danish Blue) should be avoided. However, there are so many different varieties available now that it is not always easy to know what is and isn't considered safe. Britain alone produces more than 700 cheeses, and there are many hundreds of French and Italian varieties too. It is virtually impossible to produce a list that includes every single cheese you might come across. So a guide to the different types is given here, along with some examples. This will help you understand why certain categories of cheese are best avoided. Then if you come across a cheese that isn't listed (page 69), you should be able to judge whether or not it's safe. I have included some cheeses here that aren't vegetarian, such as Parmesan and Roquefort, as women may sometimes consume them.

Hard cheeses

Cheeses such as Cheddar, Red Leicester and Parmesan-type cheeses are acidic and have a low moisture content, so they don't provide a suitable environment for bacteria to grow in. They are considered safe to eat whether they are made from pasteurised or unpasteurised milk. Crumbly hard cheeses, such as Wensleydale and Cheshire, also fall into this category.

Semi-hard cheeses

Edam and similar cheeses such as Leerdammer and Port Salut, which often have a slightly rubbery texture, are safe to eat in pregnancy.

Mould-ripened cheeses

Any cheese with a white rind, such as Brie or Camembert, should be avoided while you are pregnant. These cheeses are soft and have a relatively high moisture content, which is more suitable for bacteria to grow in, including bacteria that cause food poisoning, such as listeria. The cheeses are sprayed with *Penicillium candidum* to help them ripen from the outside. They are considered unsafe during pregnancy whether they are made from pasteurised or unpasteurised milk.

If you have a craving for this kind of cheese, all is not lost. Thorough cooking kills listeria, so it should be safe to eat these cheeses as part of a hot dish, like deep-fried Brie, or on a pizza or in a sauce. You just have to make sure they are properly cooked and piping hot all the way through.

Blue cheese

Soft blue-veined cheeses such as Roquefort and Dorset Blue Vinny should be treated the same way as the soft mould-ripened cheeses above. As they are soft, they are best avoided during pregnancy, whether made from pasteurised or unpasteurised milk, but it is safe to have them hot, for example in a hot pasta sauce or quiche.

Stilton is often included with the soft blue cheeses, but it is now considered safe during pregnancy, according to the FSA. The original advice from the Chief Medical Officer only warned against soft blue cheeses, but it was misquoted by many people, including health professionals, who advised pregnant women not to eat any blue cheese. The high salt content of Stilton and the fact that it contains little moisture makes it a low-risk food with regard to listeria.

Goats' cheese

When people talk about goats' cheese they usually mean the mould-ripened type, which has a white rind, such as Chèvre or Somerset goats' cheese. This kind of goats' cheese, like other mould-ripened cheeses, is best avoided during pregnancy because of the risk of listeria. This is true whether they are made from pasteurised or unpasteurised milk. However, they are fine if they are thoroughly cooked, so a hot tomato and goats' cheese tart is fine, as is goats' cheese on a pizza or in a quiche.

There are other types of cheese made from goats' milk which are safe to eat during pregnancy. It is fine to eat hard Cheddar-type cheeses made from goats' milk, and soft goats' cheeses if they are made from pasteurised milk and don't have a rind on, as this means they are not mould-ripened.

Soft cheeses

Cheeses such as cottage cheese, ricotta, fromage frais, mozzarella, cream cheese and processed cheese spread are all considered safe to eat during pregnancy. They have a high moisture content, but they are pasteurised and then packaged. It is best to buy these cheeses pre-packaged and make sure they are eaten before the use-by date. Avoid buying them from delicatessen counters or similar stalls where cross-contamination from other foods may occur.

CHEESES THAT ARE SAFE

Austrian smoked cheese
Babybel
Boursin
Caerphilly
Chavrie

Cheddar

Cheese spread, e.g. Dairylea, Laughing Cow, Primula

Cheestrings

Cheshire

Cottage cheese

Cream cheese, e.g. Philadelphia, or similar own-brand products often called 'soft cheese'

Double Gloucester

Edam

Emmental

Feta – bought in the UK and similar 'Greek Style cheese'

Goats' cheese – hard goats' cheese or pasteurised soft cheese without a rind

Gouda

Gruyère

Halloumi

Havarti

Jarlsberg

Lancashire

Leerdammer

Manchego

Mascarpone

Mozzarella (including unpasteurised)

Paneer

Parmesan and similar hard cheeses

Port Salut

Processed cheese

Quark

Red Leicester

Ricotta

Roulé

Smoked Applewood cheese

St Helen's Farm hard goats' cheese

Stilton

Wensleydale

NB. The rules for organic cheeses are the same as for non-organic cheeses, both for what's safe and for what to avoid.

Eggs

During pregnancy you should avoid eggs that are raw or partially cooked, as they may contain salmonella bacteria. This means you shouldn't have foods such as homemade mayonnaise and custard, which contain eggs that are not completely cooked.

However, it is safe to eat eggs that are cooked until both the white and the yolk are solid, as this will destroy any salmonella that might be present. This means you can have boiled, fried or scrambled eggs if they are cooked thoroughly. Baked foods such as cakes and biscuits are also fine. You can also have shop-bought foods such as mayonnaise, mousse and custard, which would traditionally contain raw or semi-cooked eggs, as food manufacturers make these with pasteurised egg. Pasteurisation kills any salmonella that may be present, making the food safe to eat and increasing the product's shelf-life. Supermarkets and similar shops therefore rarely, if ever, sell products containing unpasteurised eggs. You are only likely to come across products containing unpasteurised eggs if you go to a farm shop, farmers' market or specialist retailer. But even these generally pasteurise their eggs for safety.

The table shows foods that sometimes contain raw or partially cooked eggs.

Food	Safe to eat	Best avoided
Béarnaise sauce	Béarnaise sauce sold in jars at room temperature.	Homemade Béarnaise sauce, as it contains partially cooked eggs.
Biscuits, cookies	Any homemade or shop-bought.	Mixture containing raw egg, before you bake it.
Boiled eggs	Eggs boiled until the yolk and white are solid.	Soft-boiled eggs with a runny yolk.
Caesar salad	Caesar salad with shop-bought dressing.	Caesar salad with a raw egg in the dressing.
Cakes	Any homemade or shop-bought cake.	Cake mixture containing raw egg, before baking.
Carbonara	Spaghetti Carbonara ready-meal, or carbonara sauce from a shop, or homemade sauce that doesn't have raw egg.	Homemade carbonara sauce, as it contains partially cooked eggs.
Cheesecake	Any cheesecake bought from a supermarket or similar shop, as this will be made with pasteurised egg. Baked cheesecake, homemade or shop-bought.	Homemade cheesecake made with eggs but not baked in the oven.

Food	Safe to eat	Best avoided
Crème brûlée	Crème brûlée bought in a supermarket or similar shop, as this is made with pasteurised egg.	Homemade crème brûlée, as this contains partially cooked eggs.
Crème caramel	Crème caramel bought in a supermarket or similar shop, as this is made with pasteurised egg.	Homemade crème caramel, as this contains partially cooked eggs.
Custard (or crème anglaise)	Tinned custard, long-life UHT ready-made custard sold in a carton, chilled custard sold in a supermarket (even if it is labelled 'fresh custard'), custard made from powder. Custard tarts or slices sold in supermarkets or similar shops.	Homemade custard, as this contains only partially cooked eggs.
Egg nog	None.	Egg nog, in general, should be avoided, as it contains alcohol, but fresh egg nog in particular, as it contains raw eggs.
Eggs Benedict	None.	Any eggs Benedict, as the dish contains poached eggs with a soft yolk and the Hollandaise sauce may contain partially cooked eggs. ▶

Food	Safe to eat	Best avoided
Hollandaise sauce	Hollandaise sauce from a packet mix, jar or pouch bought from a supermarket or similar shop.	Homemade Hollandaise sauce, as it contains only partially cooked eggs.
Ice-cream	Any ice-cream sold pre-packaged in a tub or individually wrapped from a supermarket or similar shop.	Homemade ice-cream as it contains raw or partially cooked eggs (like custard). Soft ice-cream from an ice-cream van or kiosk as there is a risk of listeria if machinery isn't scrupulously clean.
Icing	Icing on products bought from supermarkets, bakers, coffee shops, etc. This includes hard icing, soft butter icing, icing made with cream cheese (e.g. on carrot cake) and royal icing.	Homemade royal icing as it contains raw egg white (sometimes used on wedding and Christmas cakes). The risk is very small if it has been made and stored carefully.
Lemon curd	Commercially prepared lemon curd sold in a jar and lemon curd tarts.	Homemade lemon curd, as it contains partially cooked eggs.
Marzipan	Marzipan bought in a block or on a cake (this is made without egg or with pasteurised egg). Homemade cooked marzipan, as this doesn't contain eggs.	Homemade no-cook marzipan, as it is made with raw eggs. However, if it is left to dry out on a cake for one to three days, before icing, the risk of bacterial growth is very small.

Food	Safe to eat	Best avoided
Mayonnaise	Shop-bought mayonnaise sold at room temperature (rather than chilled). Sandwiches or salads with mayonnaise bought from supermarkets or similar shops.	Homemade mayonnaise, as it contains raw eggs. Fresh mayonnaise from a farm shop or market, which is bought chilled and has a relatively soon use-by date.
Meringue	Shop-bought meringue, pavlova or lemon meringue pie. Homemade meringue that is cooked properly until solid (not sticky in the middle). This means cooking for two to three hours at 110°C, which should ensure the core temperature reaches 70°C for two minutes.	Homemade meringue that is hard on the outside but still sticky in the middle. Homemade soft meringue, such as lemon meringue pie and Baked Alaska.
Mousse	Mousse bought from a supermarket or similar shop.	Homemade mousse, as it contains raw eggs.
Omelette	Omelette cooked until all the egg is set, which means it is all cooked.	Omelette that is cooked on the outside but still runny in the centre.

▶

Food	Safe to eat	Best avoided
Quiche	Quiche bought from a supermarket should be safe to eat but it is best to heat it up and eat it hot. Homemade quiche that is cooked all the way through.	Homemade quiche that is not completely cooked and set in the centre.
Scrambled eggs	Scrambled eggs that are cooked until all the egg is set.	Scrambled egg that is still slightly runny.
Tartar sauce	Tartar sauce from a jar or sachet, as this contains pasteurised egg. Homemade tartar sauce made with hard-boiled egg yolks.	Homemade tartar sauce made with raw egg.

Eggs is eggs

Different types of chicken eggs, including organic and free-range, are just as likely to contain salmonella as standard eggs. Duck eggs have also been found with salmonella. In 2010 the FSA issued an official warning to remind people to be careful about hygiene when cooking or handling duck eggs. This was prompted by an outbreak of *Salmonella* Typhimurium DT8, linked to duck eggs, which involved 63 cases and included one death. As with chicken eggs, it is important to cook duck eggs until both the yolk and the white are solid.

British Lion Quality eggs (those stamped with a red lion) come from British hens that have been vaccinated against salmonella. They aren't guaranteed to be salmonella-free, but if you buy them from a reputable shop, store them in the fridge and eat them well before the use-by date, then the risk of salmonella is extremely small.

If you eat 'homemade' dishes containing uncooked, or partially cooked, eggs away from home, then the risk of salmonella increases. In 2007 a survey of caterers found that half didn't refrigerate their eggs and 20% of samples were older than recommended.

Peanuts

In the past, some women were told to avoid eating peanuts in pregnancy. However, this is no longer the case.

Guidelines issued in 1998 advised pregnant women with a family history of allergic conditions (including asthma and hay fever) to avoid peanuts, to reduce the risk of their baby becoming allergic to them. At the time, it was thought that soaring rates of peanut allergy might be linked to peanut consumption during pregnancy. The evidence was weak, but there was concern because of the rising number of children with this potentially life-threatening allergy. It was agreed that more research needed to be done, but in the meantime, women expecting babies most at risk were advised to avoid peanuts, as a precaution.

Now that further research has been completed, this advice has changed. More recent studies found no clear evidence that eating, or avoiding, peanuts in pregnancy had any effect on a baby's chances of developing an allergy to them. The current government advice, issued in 2009, is that if you want to eat peanuts during pregnancy, you can do so as part of a healthy, balanced diet.

Fruit and vegetables

It is important to wash all fruit and vegetables before you eat them. The idea that a bit of dirt won't do you any harm is a myth, as the outbreak of *Salmonella* Newport from lettuces in 2004 showed, along with the recent outbreak of *E. coli* associated with unwashed leeks and potatoes.

Bacteria such as *E. coli* can be found in soil, so it's important to wash any traces of dirt from the surface of fruit and vegetables. The best way to do this is to rub the food in a bowl or sink of water. Just holding it under a running tap isn't very effective and may cause bacteria to splash onto other foods or utensils. The same should be done with foods that appear clean when you buy them, such as tomatoes. Even if you aren't going to eat the skin of a fruit, it may still be a good idea to wash it. In 2012 there was an outbreak of *Salmonella* Newport linked to melon, probably because the bacteria was present on the surface of the melon, and the flesh became contaminated when it was being cut. As the skin on melon isn't eaten, you can wash it in water with washing-up liquid before cutting. It is also best to wash foods that you're going to cook, as food poisoning has been associated with foods that are always cooked, such as potatoes and leeks. It could be that bacteria are spread during food preparation via knives, chopping boards, pan handles, etc.

Although washing is enough to make most vegetables safe, this is not the case for bean sprouts. In 2010 the FSA issued a warning that bean sprouts should be thoroughly cooked before consumption, after more than 100 cases of *Salmonella* Bareilly were found with a possible link to raw bean sprouts.

Herbs

You may have heard that certain herbs, including basil, oregano, parsley, sage and thyme, should be avoided in pregnancy because they are uterine stimulants. However, it is only the essential oils, which are very concentrated and are used in aromatherapy, which could potentially cause problems. It is absolutely fine to include the herbs themselves in normal cooking.

Alcohol

The Department of Health advises pregnant women and those trying to get pregnant not to drink any alcohol. Avoiding alcohol during the first three months of pregnancy is particularly important, according to NICE, and drinking at this early stage increases the risk of miscarriage.

If you drink alcohol, it passes through the placenta from your bloodstream to your baby. Your baby can't break down alcohol as efficiently as you can, and exposure to too much alcohol can seriously effect a baby's development. It can also affect the absorption of some nutrients. If you do choose to drink alcohol, you should have no more than one to two units of alcohol once or twice a week. Also, you shouldn't get drunk or binge-drink, which is defined as having more than 7.5 units of alcohol on a single occasion. The table overleaf shows you how much alcohol different drinks contain. Remember: the advice refers to one or two *units*, not one or two *drinks*.

	Quantity	Units of alcohol
Wine		
12% ABV*	175ml glass	2
	250ml glass	3
14% ABV	250ml glass	3.5
Beer and cider		
4% ABV, e.g. Carling, Carlsberg, Fosters, Guinness, John Smiths	440ml can	2
	1 pint	2.3
4.5% ABV, e.g. Magners, Newcastle Brown, Old Speckled Hen	1 pint	2.6
5% ABV, e.g. Becks, Carlsberg Export, Heineken	275ml bottle	1.5
	1 pint	3
Alcopops		
4% ABV, e.g. Bacardi Breezer, Red Russian, Smirnoff Ice, WKD	275ml bottle	1.1
	70cl bottle	2.8
Spirits		
37.5% ABV, e.g. Smirnoff Red, Bacardi	Single (25ml)	1
	Single (35ml)	1.3
	Double (50ml)	2
	Double (70ml)	2.6

ABV is % alcohol by volume.

There is no need to count alcohol that is added to cooked dishes, such as sherry in a stir-fry or red wine in poached pears. A single portion will contain so little alcohol that it's not worth worrying about. Most recipes use very little anyway and much of the alcohol is then cooked off. It is estimated that after 15 minutes of cooking 60% of the alcohol is lost; after an hour, 75% is lost.

Heavy drinking during pregnancy (more than about 10 units a week) is associated with foetal alcohol syndrome (FAS). Babies with FAS have restricted growth and a variety of congenital abnormalities, including limb damage, heart defects and facial abnormalities. In recent years, several studies have suggested that what might be considered moderate drinking can also have adverse affects on the neurological development of some babies, resulting in learning and behavioural disorders. The term foetal alcohol syndrome disorder (FASD) is now used to describe a whole range of problems, including FAS and also less severe conditions. It is estimated that in Britain as many as one in 100 babies may be affected in some way.

Early pregnancy worries

If you drank a lot of alcohol before finding out you were pregnant, try not to worry. You're certainly not the first woman to do this and you won't be the last. There is very little chance that one or two nights of heavy drinking early on in pregnancy will cause any harm. However, once you suspect you are pregnant, it is best to be careful.

From time to time the media report on research which appears to cast doubt on the current advice, but this should be treated with caution. A study of over 11,000 UK women was reported nationally as showing that light drinking in pregnancy was better than abstinence, as it resulted in better-behaved children. What the study actually found was that drinking one or two units of alcohol a week during pregnancy didn't appear to have any negative affects on the skills that were tested. Overall, the children of light drinkers and abstainers had similar social, emotional and cognitive skills when they were five years old. They performed slightly better on some of the many tests, but this would be expected by chance. Not every aspect of development was tested, nor were long-term outcomes monitored.

The Department of Health warned that the findings were not conclusive and didn't change the advice they would be giving.

The results of studies such as this have led some experts to disagree with the government advice. They argue that there is no evidence to support a complete ban on alcohol. The problem is that the evidence is not clear-cut. Any observational survey has to rely on women's own reports about how much they have been drinking, which may not be reliable for a number of reasons. Also, women who choose to drink may have a different lifestyle from those who don't. They may be more likely to smoke or more likely to be middle-class working women with good diets, and there is no way of distinguishing which aspect of their behaviour is really affecting the health and development of their babies.

Another issue is that some babies seem to cope better with alcohol than others. The effects seem to be more severe in women with poor diets and low intakes of certain vitamins, including B vitamins. Research published at the end of 2012 suggested that the effects of alcohol on development also depend on the baby's genes. The study of more than 4,000 women who were moderate drinkers during pregnancy (1-6 units a week) looked at four genetic modifications on the genes responsible for breaking down alcohol. They found that for each genetic modification a child had, their IQ was roughly two points lower when they were eight years old. So, babies with all four genetic modifications were the least efficient at breaking down alcohol during pregnancy and their IQs were reduced by approximately eight points by moderate drinking, whereas babies with zero modifications were able to break down the same amount of alcohol without their IQ being affected.

We can't predict how an individual baby might be affected by drinking. As there is no proven safe level of exposure for a foetus, most agree that caution is the best option.

The only way to ensure a baby is not affected by alcohol is simply not to drink any.

Caffeine

Caffeine is found in coffee, tea, cola, chocolate, energy drinks such as Red Bull, and some medications such as cold and flu remedies, headache treatments and diuretics. It is a stimulant and a diuretic (it makes you wee).

It is fine to have up to 200mg of caffeine per day during pregnancy, according to the Department of Health. This is equivalent to about two cups of coffee. Having more than this can increase the risk of having a low-birth-weight baby or even a miscarriage. Caffeine crosses the placenta and affects the baby in the same way that it affects you.

One, much publicised, study carried out in the USA found that women consuming more than 200mg of caffeine a day had twice the miscarriage risk of those consuming no caffeine. Even those with low caffeine intakes were at increased risk of miscarriage compared to abstainers. On the basis of this evidence, some experts now believe it is best to avoid caffeine completely during the first 12 weeks of pregnancy, when the risk of miscarriage is highest. After that, levels below 200mg are thought to be safe.

You can use the table overleaf as a guide to help you stay within the daily limit. You could have as many as four cups of tea a day and stay within the 200mg limit, but if you like big mugs of very strong tea then you probably shouldn't have more than two a day. You could try alternatives such as decaffeinated tea or coffee, peppermint tea or fruit tea. If you occasionally have more than 200mg, don't worry too much, as the risks are likely to be very small.

	Quantity	Caffeine content (mg)
Barleycup		0
Chocolate	Plain (50g bar)	Up to 50
	Milk (50g bar)	Up to 25
	Drinking chocolate (cup)	1-8
Coffee*	Filter of percolator (cup)	100-115
	Instant (cup)	75
	Instant (mug)	100
	Espresso (single)	75-100
	Cappuccino/latte (regular)	100-200
	Americano (regular)	225-300
	Decaffeinated (mug)	3-30
Cola	Regular or diet (330ml can)	40
Energy drink	Containing caffeine or guarana (can)	Up to 80
Tea*	Medium strength (cup)	50
	Medium strength (mug)	75
	Rooibos tea	0
	Green tea (cup)	25

The amount of caffeine varies with the blend of tea leaves or coffee beans, the strength of tea or coffee and the serving size.

Guarana
This is a seed extract originally from the Amazon. It contains caffeine and related compounds and is added to some energy drinks, herbal drinks and chewing gum. It is best avoided during pregnancy and while breastfeeding as it is a stimulant and the effects on your baby are unknown.

Fruit teas and herbal teas

Fruit teas are generally considered safe for pregnancy and breastfeeding as they are made with ingredients you might normally eat, such as blackcurrant, lemon or orange. Herbal teas can be made from a variety of ingredients and it is best to avoid those made from unfamiliar ingredients, such as black cohosh, ginseng or pennyroyal. These should be treated as drugs or medicines rather than foods, as many contain active ingredients that pass through the placenta to your baby or into breast milk, in the same way that medicines do. It is best to seek professional advice regarding their safety. If you buy any kind of tea, make sure it is from a reputable source. It should come with a full list of ingredients and be labelled with the manufacturer's and distributor's details and a best-before date.

Green tea is generally regarded as being good for your health, but there is some suggestion that drinking large amounts around the time of conception may increase the risk of neural tube defects. This is because the anti-cancer compound epigallocatechin gallate (EGCG) found in green tea lowers folic acid levels. The evidence for this is far from strong, but if you are trying to get pregnant, you may want to limit your intake to no more than about two cups a day.

Peppermint tea and ginger tea are safe to take during pregnancy and some women find they help relieve morning sickness, nausea and digestive problems. There is some suggestion, although no real evidence, that drinking large quantities of peppermint tea could cause miscarriage. As a precaution, you may want to avoid drinking several strong cups of peppermint tea close together. There is also some concern over the safety of drinking fennel tea during pregnancy; again there is no real evidence but you might want to avoid it. Raspberry leaf tea is a uterine stimulant and should be avoided until the later stages of pregnancy (see page 161). If you are breastfeeding, then teas made with fennel, fenugreek, aniseed, raspberry leaf and nettle are thought to increase milk supply. Sage tea is sometimes used to reduce milk production and women may take it when they decide to stop breastfeeding.

Buying and preparing safe food

As you are more susceptible to food poisoning while you are pregnant, it's important to pay special attention to food hygiene. There is usually a delay between eating contaminated food and the first signs of a problem. This is known as the incubation period and it can range from a few hours to several days, depending on the bacteria's method of attack. Some bacteria stick to the lining of the intestine and destroy cells directly. These cause symptoms such as nausea, vomiting, abdominal cramps and diarrhoea. Others produce a toxin that is absorbed and can produce symptoms such as headaches. In warm environments bacteria can multiply rapidly, for example at picnics and barbecues and on buffet tables. In such environments, a single bacterium can become several million bacteria within about eight hours.

You can reduce your risks of getting food poisoning considerably by taking some sensible precautions when you are preparing and storing food, and when you eat out or get a take-away. In the USA, Australia and New Zealand, pregnant women are advised to avoid buying food from delicatessen counters. In the UK there are no specific guidelines about deli foods, but it may be safer to stick to pre-packaged foods wherever possible. When foods aren't packaged, cross-contamination from one food to another can occur and use-by dates may not be followed strictly. Other potential concerns are foods and drinks bought from market stalls or street sellers that you are going to consume cold, such as freshly squeezed orange juice and slices of melon.

Preparing food

- Always wash your hands before eating or preparing food.
- Wash all fruit and vegetables before eating, including bags of salad leaves labelled as 'washed and ready to eat'.
- Wash your hands, knife and chopping board after preparing unwashed vegetables, before going on to prepare foods to be eaten raw (otherwise traces of soil can be transferred and eaten).
- Keep your kitchen clean and don't allow pets on tables or kitchen work surfaces.
- Before eating hot foods, make sure they are piping hot all the way through. This is particularly important for foods such as ready-meals and pies.
- When microwaving food, follow the instructions carefully, including stirring and standing times. Then check the food is cooked all the way through before eating it.
- If you handle raw eggs, wash your hands, utensils and any spillages thoroughly with hot soapy water, otherwise bacteria can spread to fridge handles, cutlery and other foods.
- While you're cooking, you shouldn't taste anything containing raw eggs, such as cake mixture or cookie dough, before it's been cooked. Cookie dough ice-cream from a shop is fine, however, as it is made with pasteurised egg.

Storing food

- Make sure the temperature of your fridge is below 5°C and that of your freezer is below -18°C.

- Don't eat anything beyond its 'use by' date, even if it looks and smells fine. As food prices have risen sharply, more people are doing this, but bugs like *E. coli* and salmonella can reach dangerous levels without affecting the smell or taste of a food. When it comes to 'best before' dates, these aren't related to safety but to quality, so you can use your own judgement.

- Store raw eggs in the fridge away from other foods and bear in mind that salmonella can be present on eggshells.

- Cool and refrigerate any leftovers within an hour of cooking and eat them within 24 hours.

Risky rice

Take particular care with left-over rice, rice salads and dishes containing re-heated rice, such as kedgeree, biryani and egg-fried rice. Rice can contain spores of *Bacillus cereus* bacteria, which can germinate if the dish is left standing at room temperature. The longer the rice is left, the more these bacteria will multiply. The bacteria produce toxins that can cause food poisoning (vomiting and diarrhoea). It is not known whether there are any other effects during pregnancy. Once cooked, rice should be eaten hot, or cooled down and put in the fridge within an hour. It should then be eaten within 24 hours or thrown away.

Take-aways and eating out

When someone else is preparing your food, it is impossible to be 100% sure about hygiene standards. It is best to eat only in places you trust, and it is generally safer to choose hot dishes rather than cold ones such as salads. If you get a take-away meal and it isn't piping hot when it arrives, you could heat it in the microwave as an extra precaution.

Don't be afraid to ask about ingredients or information about how a dish has been prepared, for example whether it contains homemade mayonnaise. Most places will be happy to help, and a bit of embarrassment now is better than worrying about something later.

Different types of food poisoning

Campylobacter

Campylobacter is the most common bacterial cause of food poisoning in the UK. Every year around 50,000 to 60,000 cases are reported to the Health Protection Agency. Although it is mainly found in meat and poultry, unpasteurised milk and untreated water can also be infected.

Infection with campylobacter doesn't usually result in vomiting, but symptoms can be very severe and include fever, abdominal cramps and diarrhoea, which may contain blood. Infection during pregnancy can result in premature delivery or miscarriage. But if the infection is detected, then intravenous antibiotic treatment can be given.

Listeria

Listeria (*Listeria monocytogenes*) is a type of bacteria found in some foods, soil, vegetation and sewage. It can cause an illness called listeriosis, which can have serious consequences during pregnancy. It is impossible to tell whether a food is contaminated with listeria as it will look, smell and taste normal. Listeria is found in small amounts in many foods, but some, such as ready-meals, may have much higher levels.

Pregnant women are about 20 times more likely than other adults to get listeriosis, because of hormonal changes affecting their immune system. Although the illness is unlikely to be serious for the mother, it can result in miscarriage, premature delivery, stillbirth or severe illness in newborn babies. The number of cases of food poisoning from listeriosis have increased considerably since 2000 and, although it is still fairly rare, you can reduce your risks further by following the general rules about hygiene and avoiding the following foods:

- Soft mould-ripened cheeses and soft blue-veined cheeses (see page 68).
- Pâté, including all vegetable pâtés.
- Unpasteurised dairy products, including milk, cream, yogurt and ice-cream.
- Pre-packaged salad leaves – unless they are washed thoroughly.
- Ready-meals such as curry and lasagne – unless they are re-heated carefully following the manufacturer's guidelines so that they are piping hot all the way through.

The FSA is currently reviewing its advice about listeria and which foods pregnant women should avoid and it is possible that this list may change slightly in the future.

Symptoms of listeriosis can take between three and 70 days to appear after exposure and may include fever, a mild flu-like illness or diarrhoea. These symptoms can, of course, have other causes. If you are concerned, it is best to talk to your GP, who may ask for blood or urine tests. If you do have listeriosis, it can usually be treated successfully with antibiotics.

Toxoplasmosis

This is an infection caused by a microscopic parasite called *Toxoplasmosis gondii*. More than half of people with toxoplasmosis don't know they have it, but in others It can cause flu-like symptoms or more severe symptoms similar to those of glandular fever. If a woman becomes infected during pregnancy or in the two to three months before conception, it can cause miscarriage, stillbirth or a range of birth defects, including hydrocephalus ('water on the brain'), brain damage, epilepsy, deafness, blindness or growth problems.

Meat is responsible for most cases of toxoplasmosis but it can also be caused by unpasteurised milk or milk products and any food contaminated with soil. As well as making sure that fruit and vegetables are completely free of soil, women are advised to wear gloves when gardening and handling cat litter, and to wash their hands carefully afterwards.

If you think you may have toxoplasmosis, it is important to see your doctor. You can have blood tests; if these are positive, then your baby can also be tested via amniocentesis. In about 40% of toxoplasmosis cases, the infection is passed from a mother to her baby. However, if the mother is treated promptly with antibiotics, it can prevent her baby from becoming infected. If the baby is already infected, then different antibiotics can be given to reduce the severity of the infection.

Salmonella

This is one of the most common causes of food poisoning. It differs from the listeria and toxoplasmosis bugs because it doesn't cross the placenta to the foetus. However, salmonella can make you very ill, with a high temperature that could harm your baby. Symptoms include heavy vomiting and diarrhoea, but the effects vary. There are 200 different strains of salmonella. High-risk foods include raw or partially cooked eggs (see page 71).

Brucella

This bacteria is sometimes found in unpasteurised milk and dairy products, including cheeses and yogurt. Infection can result in fever, illness and miscarriage. It is rare in the UK but more common in Middle Eastern countries and some Mediterranean countries, including Spain. If you are travelling abroad it is best to ensure that any dairy products are made from pasteurised milk. At home, avoid 'country' or 'locally made' cheeses from other countries.

E. coli

Most strains of *Escherichia coli* (*E. coli*) bacteria are harmless, but some can cause severe food poisoning. These are verocytoxin-producing *E. coli* (VTECs). In the UK EO157 is the most common VTEC, but in other countries EO111 and EO26 are more common. Harmful strains of *E. coli* may be found in unpasteurised milk or transmitted directly from infected animals, people and soil. In 2011 there was an outbreak of *E. coli* O157 in England involving 250 people. It was found that the outbreak was associated with handling loose unwashed vegetables, including leeks and potatoes.

If a pregnant woman contracts *E. coli*, it isn't transmitted to the foetus. However, symptoms can be serious and include bloody diarrhoea and abdominal cramps. The illness can also have serious complications, such as severe anaemia and problems with the nervous system and kidneys.

6 Getting enough iron and avoiding anaemia

Iron deficiency isn't uncommon during pregnancy, whether you're vegetarian or not. Iron's main role in the body is in the formation of healthy red blood cells, which carry oxygen around the body. It is also needed for the production of several enzymes, including some of those involved in digestion and the normal functioning of the liver and nervous system. During pregnancy, you need more iron than usual. It is used to build your baby and placenta, but also to produce extra red blood cells for you and to help your body cope with losing blood during delivery.

One of the many amazing things your body does during pregnancy is to adapt its digestive system to become much more efficient at absorbing iron from the food you eat. Usually humans absorb less than 20% of the iron they consume in food. However, in the second trimester of pregnancy, iron absorption increases by about 50%. In the last trimester, you absorb about four times as much of the iron you consume. Because of this increase in efficiency, pregnant women aren't advised to consume any more iron than non-pregnant women. Unfortunately this doesn't mean you can simply ignore your iron intake, because most women consume less iron than is recommended.

Pregnant women generally have a blood sample taken at the first appointment with their midwife and this is used to test for iron levels, among other things. If the blood tests show you are anaemic or iron deficient, your midwife will let you know and will probably prescribe iron supplements (see page 99).

Signs of iron deficiency are as follows:

- Feeling especially weak or tired and lethargic.
- Shortness of breath.
- Dizziness or fainting.
- Headaches.
- Feeling more irritable than usual.
- Pica (a craving for chalk, mud or any other non-foodstuffs).
- Restless Leg Syndrome (page 155).
- Feeling colder than normal.

Having low iron levels also has more serious consequences during pregnancy. It is linked to lower birth weight, prematurity, pre-eclampsia, increased risk of haemorrhage and postnatal depression. A lack of iron is also associated with developmental delays, as iron is particularly important for the development of your baby's brain. Also, if you are iron deficient during pregnancy there is a greater risk that your baby will be born iron deficient.

Are you getting enough iron?

During pregnancy you need about 14.8mg of iron per day. A recent study carried out among more than 1,200 pregnant women in the Leeds area found that only 20% managed to achieve this. The study included more than 100 vegetarians, and interestingly it was found that these women were slightly more likely than the non-vegetarians to be getting enough iron from their food. The vegetarians were also more likely to take a supplement containing iron. Perhaps this was due to the common belief that vegetarians are more likely to be anaemic. Interestingly, vegans have been found to have higher iron intakes than lacto-ovo-vegetarians, because dairy products are low in iron.

The only indicator you really have of whether you are getting enough iron is the result of your blood tests, and whether you have a low haemoglobin (Hb) and Mean Cell Volume (MCV). However, mild iron deficiency can affect health even if you're not officially anaemic. Also, these tests aren't usually done until the end of the first trimester, and it is important to have a good iron intake from as early as possible in pregnancy. The table overleaf will help you estimate whether you're getting enough iron and see how you can boost your intake. It really is worth trying to get the iron you need from food rather than supplements, as iron supplements are often poorly absorbed and can cause other problems such as constipation, as well as reducing absorption of other minerals.

While vegetarians are no more likely than meat-eaters to have anaemia, several studies have shown they have lower iron stores. During pregnancy most women have their serum ferritin levels measured, which is an indicator of iron stores. If your ferritin level is found to be low, you may not even be told about it, or you may be prescribed iron supplements. It depends on how important individual care providers think this is. Having low iron stores isn't a problem in itself, but it means you're more likely to develop anaemia. Look at your antenatal notes and if you find your ferritin level is low then you should be particularly vigilant, and ensure you get plenty of iron in your diet (serum ferritin below 12µg/L is generally considered low but this varies between hospitals).

Where is iron found?

Iron is found in a wide variety of foods and comes in two different forms. Haem iron is present in meat and fish, and is absorbed by the body more easily than non-haem iron, which comes from plant sources. This is sometimes used as an argument to show that diets including meat are superior. However, generally no more than about 10% of the average meat-eater's iron comes in the form of haem iron; the remaining 90% is non-haem iron. In the Leeds study mentioned earlier, it was found that only 5% of the pregnant women's iron intake came from meat and fish. That said, vegetarians do need to think about including good sources of iron in their diet every day.

Food	Iron (mg) per 100g	Iron per portion
Breakfast cereals		
Muesli	5.8	2.9mg per 50g
Porridge oats	4.1	2.0mg per 50g
Wheats, e.g. Shredded Wheat	4.2	1.8mg per two bisks
Wheat bisks, e.g. Weetabix*	11.9	4.5mg per two bisks
Special K and similar*	11.6–22.0	4.6–9.0mg per 40g
Bran flakes*	11.6–14.0	4.5–5.6mg per 40g
Cornflakes*	8.0–14.0	3.2–5.6mg per 40g
Instant hot oats*	11.9	4.8mg per 40g
Starchy foods		
White bread	1.7	1.2mg per two slices
Wholemeal bread	2.4	1.8mg per two slices
White pasta (cooked)	0.5	1.1mg per 220g
Wholemeal pasta (cooked)	1.1	2.4mg per 220g
White rice (cooked)	0.2	0.4mg per 100g
Brown rice (cooked)	0.5	1.0mg per 200g
Potatoes	0.4	0.8mg per 200g

Food	Iron (mg) per 100g	Iron per portion
Pulses and vegetables		
Lentils (cooked)	3.5	2.8mg per 2 tablespoons
Chickpeas (cooked)	2.1	1.4mg per 2 tablespoons
Kidney beans (cooked)	2.5	1.7mg per 2 tablespoons
Baked beans	1.4	2.8mg per half-tin (200g)
Spinach (cooked)	1.6	1.3mg per 80g
Broccoli (cooked)	1.0	0.8mg per 80g
Peas (cooked)	1.6	1.3mg per 80g
Other foods		
Eggs	1.9	1.2mg per egg
Houmous	1.9	1.0mg per 2 tablespoons
Tahini	10.6	2.0mg per heaped teaspoon
Dried apricots	4.1	1mg per five fruits
Raisins	3.8	1.1mg per tablespoon

These cereals are usually fortified; unfortified varieties contain less iron.

Source: Data taken from various sources including the UK Nutrient Databank © Crown copyright 2012

Another way of increasing the amount of iron in your diet is by cooking in cast iron cookware. This isn't very common in the UK, but balti curries are traditionally cooked in iron woks and even supermarket-bought vegetable baltis have been found to have a much higher iron content than other vegetable curries. The iron accumulated during cooking also seems to be quite well absorbed, so you might want to think about investing in a cast-iron cooking pot.

Guinness and spinach for iron power?

Guinness and other stouts were once thought to be good for pregnancy because they contained lots of iron and would 'build you up'. However, Guinness contains approximately 0.01mg of iron per 100ml, or 0.3mg per half-pint. A typical bowl of breakfast cereal contains about 10 times as much (3.0–7.0mg per bowl). Stout also contains alcohol, of course, which isn't good for pregnancy or breastfeeding.

You might also be advised to eat spinach for extra iron. If this is what Popeye was relying on, he was mistaken. Although spinach does contain iron, it also has high levels of oxalic acid, which binds tightly to the iron, so it can't be absorbed. This means the iron in spinach is likely to pass straight through the body.

Tips for boosting your iron absorption

The amount of iron we absorb from our food varies between about 1% and 30%. It depends to a large extent on the other nutrients and phytochemicals present in a meal. To increase absorption:

- Have vitamin C at the same time as iron-rich foods, for example a glass of orange juice with your breakfast cereal, broccoli with stir-fried tofu, or strawberries after beans on toast.

- Avoid tea, coffee and cocoa for an hour either side of meals. The polyphenols in these drinks reduce iron absorption.

- When you have an iron-rich food such as lentils, don't always have it with wholegrain products such as wholewheat pasta or brown rice. These high-fibre foods contain phytate, which binds to iron, so less is absorbed.
- Have sourdough bread. The phytate level is reduced when the dough is fermented, so the absorption of iron and other minerals is improved.

Iron supplements

You will need to take iron supplements during pregnancy only if blood tests show that you have low levels of iron. Depending on how low your haemoglobin (Hb) level is, you may be advised to take a supplement containing between 100mg and 200mg. In some countries, including the USA and France, women are routinely advised to take iron supplements, but in the UK it is argued that if your iron levels are normal then taking high doses of iron may actually be harmful. However, it's still fine to take a multivitamin and mineral supplement containing iron, as it will have a much lower dose – around 15mg.

The best way to take iron supplements
- Take your supplement on an empty stomach, an hour before a meal.
- Have a glass of orange juice at the same time to increase absorption.
- Don't have tea, coffee or prune juice with your supplement.
- Don't take other medicines, supplements or antacids at the same time.

Some women find that taking the prescribed supplements, which are usually ferrous sulphate, causes unpleasant side effects such as nausea and constipation. This is more likely to be the case if you're taking more than 100mg of ferrous iron per day. If you do have problems then it may help if you take a lower dose, take supplements only every other day, or take them with meals. Ideally, supplements shouldn't be taken with food, because the iron interferes with the absorption of other minerals such as zinc, but it's better than not taking the supplements because they make you feel awful.

Alternatively, you could switch to a different iron supplement. Talk to your GP or midwife first, as they may be able to offer iron in a different form, for example iron gluconate. Or you could choose a supplement yourself, such as Spatone™, which appears to cause fewer side effects but can still be effective in treating anaemia. The downside of choosing a different supplement is that you'll have to pay for it yourself – though if it makes you feel better, it's generally worth it.

Cord clamping

When your baby is born the umbilical cord will be clamped and cut, and the timing of this can have a significant effect on the baby's iron levels. In the past the umbilical cord was usually clamped straight away after a baby was delivered. It was thought that delaying this beyond about 30 seconds would increase the risk of the baby developing jaundice and the mother haemorrhaging after delivery. Newer research shows this isn't the case. Another reason given for clamping sooner rather than later was that it protected the baby from being exposed to the hormones given to the mother to speed up labour and delivery of the placenta.

However, it has been found that a newborn's blood volume can be boosted by a third if the cord isn't clamped for three minutes after birth and the baby remains connected to the mother's blood supply. As a result, delaying clamping reduces the risk of iron deficiency and anaemia in the baby. It also allows the transfer of vital stem cells.

Due to growing evidence that the benefits of delayed clamping outweigh the drawbacks, the Royal College of Midwives published new guidelines at the end of 2012. Midwives are now encouraged to clamp the umbilical cord three to five minutes after delivery. As this advice was issued relatively recently, some midwives may not be in the habit of delaying clamping, so you might want to talk to your midwife about it and maybe put it into your birth plan. Bear in mind that delaying clamping isn't always possible, for example if the baby needs immediate support or the cord is around the baby's neck and needs to be cut straight away. Also, when a baby is born prematurely or by caesarean, it may be better to cut the cord earlier than three minutes after delivery. However, for the majority of babies it now seems that delaying clamping is the best option.

7 Other essential vitamins and minerals

Iron receives a lot of attention during pregnancy, but there are several other vitamins and minerals that are also essential for a healthy pregnancy, including vitamin B_{12} and iodine. While iron levels are routinely checked with blood tests, levels of these other nutrients aren't monitored, so it's important to become as knowledgeable about them as possible to ensure a good intake.

There are two types of vitamins: water-soluble and fat-soluble. The water-soluble vitamins are the B vitamins and vitamin C. These are easily lost if foods are overcooked or boiled in lots of water that is then thrown away. Water-soluble vitamins are also lost more easily from the body. So, if you have an excess intake of vitamin C, it is passed out in your urine. However, with fat-soluble vitamins (A, D and E), you have to be careful not to have too much, as these aren't excreted as easily.

Vitamin A

What it's for: This vitamin is needed for a strong immune system and the development of healthy skin and eyes. One of the first signs of vitamin A deficiency is night blindness, which is an inability to see in dim light. More severe deficiency can result in permanent eye damage. It is also important for the development of your baby's lungs.

Amount needed: During pregnancy you need about 700µg of vitamin A (retinol equivalents[1]) per day. This increases to 950µg per day while breastfeeding.

Where it's found: There are two forms of vitamin A: retinol and beta-carotene. Retinol is found in animal products, including eggs and milk, and beta-carotene is found in carrots and other orange fruit and vegetables.

	Vitamin A (µg) per 100g[*]	*Vitamin A per portion*
Milk	25	75µg per half-pint/300ml
Eggs	190	110µg per egg
Carrots	2,230	1,780µg per 80g portion
Mango	116	19µg per 80g portion
Apricots	68	100µg per three apricots
Cantaloupe melon	283	435µg per 150g slice

[*]*1ug of beta-carotene has the effect of approximately 6ug of retinol. The vitamin A content of the foods containing beta-carotene is given here as retinol equivalents. They don't contain any retinol, but this allows direct comparison with the level of vitamin A that is recommended.*

Source: Data taken from the UK Nutrient Databank © Crown copyright 2012

High intakes: Although you need some vitamin A, if you have too much, the levels in your body can build up, which can be a problem. Vitamin A in the form of retinol is teratogenic – a high intake (more than about 3,300µg per day) is associated with an increase in birth defects. This is why pregnant women should avoid liver, fish liver oils (e.g. cod liver oil) and other supplements containing large amounts of retinol. It is perfectly safe to eat other foods containing retinol, such as milk and eggs, as they contain less than 1% of the concentration found in liver. You can also eat foods containing beta-carotene without worrying; the worst effect this could have is to make your skin look slightly orange. Some experts believe that women need to increase their intake of beta-carotene during pregnancy, as vitamin A deficiency can be a real risk, particularly in women having twins or having babies close together.

Folic acid

What it's for: Folic acid is one of the B vitamins and reduces the risk of your baby developing a neural tube defect, such as spina bifida. It also reduces the risk of cleft palate and harelip, and it works with vitamin B_{12} to form healthy red blood cells.

Amount needed: Women who aren't pregnant or planning to have a baby need 200µg of folic acid per day. This increases to 300µg a day during pregnancy and 260µg per day if you are breastfeeding. You should also take a folic acid supplement before pregnancy and for the first 12 weeks (see page 134). Vegetarians have higher folic acid intakes than non-vegetarians, but supplements are recommended for everyone, as it is almost impossible to get enough folic acid, in a form that is easily absorbed, from food alone.

Where it's found: Folic acid is found naturally as folate in many fruits and vegetables. However, it is easily lost. For example, frozen peas contain 78μg of folate per 100g, but if you boil them in a pan of water this goes down to just 33μg per 100g. To preserve the folate, it is best to microwave, steam, cook in small amounts of water or add vegetables to dishes such as curry, where there is no cooking water to throw away. Folic acid is also added to many processed foods including some breakfast cereals, bread and yeast extract. Different brands are fortified with different amounts.

	Folate (μg) per 100g	Folate per portion
Broccoli	75	60μg per 80g portion
Peas	55	44μg per 80g portion
Oranges	31	50μg per medium orange
Milk	8	25μg per half-pint/ 300ml
Marmite	2,500	100μg per 4g portion
Vegemite	2,000	80μg per 4g portion
Fruit and fibre cereal	125–250	50–100μg per 40g bowl
Bran flakes	300–400	120–160μg per 40g bowl
Oatmeal	60	30μg per 50g portion

Source: Data taken from various sources including the UK Nutrient Databank © Crown copyright 2012

Vitamin B_2 (riboflavin)

What it's for: Riboflavin is needed for the conversion of fats, protein and carbohydrate into energy. Deficiency can result in cracked skin at the corners of the mouth and skin problems around the nose, eyes and tongue.

Amount needed: You need 1.4mg per day during pregnancy and 1.6mg per day while breastfeeding. If you consume too much it will be excreted in your urine.

Where it's found: It is found in a wide variety of foods.

	Riboflavin (mg) per 100g	Riboflavin per portion
Milk	0.2	0.6mg per half-pint/ 300ml
Cheddar	0.4	0.1mg per 30g portion
Mushrooms	0.3	0.2mg per 80g portion
Almonds	0.75	0.2mg per 25g handful
Marmite	7.0	0.3mg per 4g portion
Vegemite	8.6	0.3mg per 4g portion
Weetabix and similar cereals	1.2	0.5mg per two bisks

Source: Data taken from various sources including the UK Nutrient Databank © Crown copyright 2012

Vitamin B$_6$ (pyridoxine)

What it's for: Vitamin B$_6$ is needed for the metabolism of protein and the release of energy from foods. It is also required for the development of a healthy nervous system and red blood cells. Deficiency is rare, but there is some evidence that women with low levels are less likely to become pregnant and more likely to miscarry in early pregnancy. There is also some evidence that low levels are linked with morning sickness. Vitamin B$_6$ supplements are sometimes used to treat hyperemisis gravidarum (see page 134).

Amount needed: You need about 1.2mg per day. There is no extra requirement for pregnancy or breastfeeding.

Where it's found: It is found in nuts and some fruit and vegetables, especially potatoes if you eat the skin too. It is also found in fish.

	Vitamin B$_6$ (mg) per 100g	Vitamin B$_6$ per portion
Nuts (hazelnuts, peanuts, walnuts)	0.59–0.67	0.2mg per 30g handful
Bananas	0.29	0.3mg per medium banana
Avocados	0.36	0.3mg per half avocado
Red peppers	0.36	0.2mg per half pepper
Potatoes	0.54	1.0mg per potato with skin
Wholemeal bread	0.11	0.1mg per two slices
Tofu	0.09	0.1mg per portion (quarter-block)
Milk	0.06	0.2mg per half-pint

Source: Data taken from the UK Nutrient Databank © Crown copyright 2012

Vitamin B$_{12}$

What it's for: This vitamin is important for healthy red blood cells, the release of energy from food, and the development and normal functioning of the nervous system. It is also necessary for the body to be able to process folic acid. Women with low vitamin B$_{12}$ levels appear to be at greater risk of pregnancy complications, including neural tube defects. However, evidence for this is only limited, compared with the very strong evidence of association between folic acid and spina bifida prevention. Research with pregnant Dutch women found those with low vitamin B$_{12}$ levels in early pregnancy were more likely to have babies who were colicky and cried for three or more hours a day.

Amount needed: The official UK recommendations are for 1.5µg of vitamin B_{12} per day during pregnancy and 2.0µg per day while breastfeeding. However, other countries, including the US and Norway, recommend higher intakes, and the UK advice may change in the future. To be on the safe side you should aim for at least 3µg per day. As it is best absorbed in small amounts, it is better if this is spread out throughout the day. If you are getting all your vitamin B_{12} at one time by taking a daily supplement then a higher dose may be better; the Vegan Society advise 10µg per day if you're getting all your vitamin B_{12} from a daily supplement.

As it is found naturally only in foods of animal origin, vegetarians tend to have a lower intake. In a study of pregnant women in the Netherlands it was found that lacto-ovo-vegetarians were more likely to be vitamin B_{12} deficient than other women. Blood tests showed that 22% of lacto-ovo-vegetarians were vitamin B_{12} deficient, compared with 10% of 'low-meat-eaters' and 3% of non-vegetarians. There have also been a number of cases of severe vitamin B_{12} deficiency among vegans who were breastfeeding and their babies.

Where it's found: It is found in almost all foods of animal origin but in virtually no foods of plant origin. Most soya milks are fortified, but organic soya milks are not allowed to be fortified, so they don't contain any vitamin B_{12}. Some other milk-alternatives are also fortified, including Oatly Oat Drink but not Rice Dream original nor Kara Coconut milk. Some breakfast cereals are also fortified with B_{12}, but again, others are not. More natural cereals, such as muesli and porridge oats, don't contain any vitamin B_{12} but bran flakes and cornflakes do (unless you buy organic). Yeast extract is often recommended as a good source of vitamin B_{12} for vegans, but it's worth noting that while Marmite and most supermarket own brands of yeast extract have added vitamin B$_{12}$, Vegemite doesn't. The real message is that if you're vegan, or don't have milk or eggs daily, you have to read the label to see which food and drink products have it added, and include these as a regular part of your diet. One easy way to boost your intake is to use a fortified yeast extract in cooking. A spoonful can be used instead of stock in dishes like pasta sauce or chilli.

	Vitamin B$_{12}$ (µg) per 100g	Vitamin B$_{12}$ per portion
Milk	0.8-1.0	2.5µg per half-pint/300ml
Yogurt (plain)	0.3	0.4µg per small pot
Eggs	1.1	1.2µg per two eggs
Soya milk-alternative (Alpro original)*	0.4	1.2µg per half-pint/300ml
Oat milk-alternative (Oatly)*	0.4	1.2µg per half-pint/300ml
Soya desserts/ custard (Alpro)*	0.4	0.5µg per small pot
Pure dairy-free soya spread (margarine substitute)*	5.0	0.5µg per 10g serving
Marmite (Vegemite has no vitamin B$_{12}$ added)*	15	0.6µg per 4g serving
Shreddies*	1.6	0.6µg per 40g bowl
Bran flakes (various brands)*	1.0-2.5	0.4-1.0µg per 40g bowl

*These figures are correct at the time of writing but manufacturers may change product ingredients, so it is best to check food labels.

Source: Data taken from various sources including the UK Nutrient Databank © Crown copyright 2012

Some people believe that certain foods made from fermented soya beans, such as tempeh and miso, as well as some sea vegetables, are good sources of vitamin B_{12}. Chemical tests have shown that these do indeed contain the vitamin. However, more complex analysis has shown that up to 90% of the vitamin found in them is an inactive analogue, which means the body can't use it. It is much better for vegans to rely on fortified foods or supplements for vitamin B_{12}.

Choline

This is not by strict definition a vitamin, although it is sometimes grouped with the B vitamins. Choline is important for fat metabolism and the transmission of nerve impulses. There is also some evidence that choline plays a role in memory. The main sources of choline for lacto-ovo-vegetarians are milk and eggs. It is also found at lower levels in many plant-derived foods. The best sources appear to be soya milk, tofu, cauliflower and broccoli. The body can make small amounts of choline, but not enough for optimal health. Individual requirements appear to vary according to genetic makeup. It is thought that additional choline is required during pregnancy, but you should be able to get an adequate amount through a varied diet.

Vitamin C (ascorbic acid)

What it's for: This vitamin protects cells and keeps them healthy. Vitamin C is particularly important for wound healing. It also increases the absorption of iron from foods of plant origin, such as breakfast cereals, bread, beans and vegetables.

Amount needed: During pregnancy, 50mg is needed per day. This increases to 70mg per day while breastfeeding. Most vegetarians meet or exceed the requirement if they have a good diet, including a variety of fruit and vegetables. As low iron levels can be a particular problem during pregnancy, it's a good idea to eat vitamin C-rich foods at the same time as iron-rich foods (see page 98).

Where it's found: Citrus fruits are the best-known source. Eating a single orange will provide more than enough vitamin C for the day. It is also found in other fruits and a wide variety of vegetables. As vitamin C is lost easily, it is best to steam or lightly cook vegetables, or add them to dishes such as curry or soup. Research carried out in China has shown that when broccoli is steamed, the vitamin C content is virtually unchanged, whereas microwaving or stir-frying broccoli reduces levels by about a fifth. Boiling broccoli had the biggest affect, with a third or more of the vitamin C lost. Once fruit is cut, the vitamin C level starts to decrease too, so it's best to eat cut fruit as soon as possible.

	Vitamin C (mg) per 100g	Vitamin C per portion
Oranges	54	86mg per medium orange
Strawberries	77	61mg per 80g portion
Kiwi fruit	59	35mg per kiwi
Potatoes (boiled, chips, etc.)	8-10	12-15mg per portion
Crisps	35	10mg per 30g bag
Broccoli (raw)	87	70mg per 80g portion
Cauliflower (raw)	43	34mg per 80g portion
Red pepper (raw)	140	42mg per quarter pepper

Source: Data taken from the UK Nutrient Databank © Crown copyright 2012

Vitamin D

What it's for: This vitamin helps with absorption of calcium and building strong, healthy bones. It is particularly important during the later stages of pregnancy. If you don't get enough vitamin D during pregnancy or while breastfeeding, your baby will have low vitamin D and calcium levels. This can lead to the baby developing seizures in the first months of life. It also puts the baby at risk of developing the bone disease rickets, which results in a softening of the bones as they grow and is characterised by bowed legs. Other symptoms of deficiency in babies are poor teeth formation and general ill health. Not getting enough vitamin D during pregnancy could also mean your baby's bone mass is lower than it should be in childhood, which means an increased risk of osteoporosis in later life. Recent research also suggests that a lack of vitamin D in pregnancy may also increase the risks of the baby developing multiple sclerosis.

Amount needed: Most adults can get enough vitamin D from a healthy diet and normal exposure to the sun. However, over recent years there has been increasing concern over vitamin D deficiency. Ultraviolet B (UVB) radiation converts a vitamin D precursor in the skin to the active form of the vitamin. People with darker skins are at greater risk of deficiency, as they require longer exposure to sunlight to make the same amount of vitamin D. This means women with darker skin are at greater risk of deficiency than those with paler skin. Women who have limited exposure to sunlight are also more likely to be deficient in vitamin D, for example those who remain covered for religious reasons when they go outside, and shift workers. Women who are pregnant or breastfeeding require extra vitamin D and should take a supplement (see page 135).

During the summer months, about 15 minutes of sunlight on the hands and face every day will supply enough vitamin D. But in winter, people living at latitudes above 52 degrees (in the UK that means north of Birmingham) are thought to receive no light of the appropriate wavelength to make vitamin D in their skin. This means they have to rely on food and supplements to meet their vitamin D needs. Research has shown that lacto-ovo-vegetarians have lower levels of vitamin D in their blood than non-vegetarians, and vegans have lower levels still.

Where it's found: Very few foods contain vitamin D naturally and most that do are unsuitable for vegans. All margarines in the UK have had vitamin D added to them since 1940, when there were worries over the nation's poor intake. The regulations don't apply to other spreads, such as reduced-fat spreads, but most still have added vitamin D anyway. A growing number of other foods also have vitamin D added, including some (but not all) probiotic drinks, breakfast cereals and soya products.

Two different forms of vitamin D are used for fortification: ergocalciferol (vitamin D2) and cholecalciferol (vitamin D3). Vitamin D2 is usually derived from yeast. It is considered acceptable for vegans and it is often added to soya products and milk-alternatives made from soya, oats or hemp. Vitamin D3 is usually derived from sheep's wool and is not approved by the Vegan Society. However, the Vegetarian Society approves foods with vitamin D3 added if the D3 is extracted from the wool of live sheep and not after slaughter. Vitamin D3 (from live sheep) is used to fortify some breakfast cereals (including some Kellogg's products) as well as most margarines and spreads. Many fortified foods just list 'vitamin D' on the label without specifying whether they use D2 or D3, but D3 from live sheep is quite widely used. If you are a vegan and want to find out, you can contact manufacturers. Some vegans decide that eating foods with D3 added is a compromise they're willing to make. Vitamin D2 has been shown in some trials to be much less potent than D3, but this may just be when the immediate response in considered. In the longer term, the two may not be quite so different.

	Vitamin D (µg) per 100g	Vitamin D per portion
Eggs	1.8	1µg per egg
Margarines	7.5	0.8µg per 10g serving
Milk	Just a trace	Just a trace
Soya milk with added vitamin D (e.g. Alpro original, Sainsbury's, Tesco)*	0.8	2.4µg per half-pint/ 300ml
Organic soya milk	0	0
Alpro desserts*	0.8	1µg per 125g pot
Cereals fortified with vitamin D (e.g. Kellogg's bran flakes, Ready Brek, Sainsbury's cornflakes)*	4–5	1.6–2µg per 40g bowl
Cereals not fortified with vitamin D (e.g. Kellogg's cornflakes, muesli, Weetabix, Shreddies)*	0	0

*These figures are correct at the time of writing but manufacturers may change product ingredients, so it is best to check food labels.

Source: Data taken from various sources including the UK Nutrient Databank © Crown copyright 2012

Vitamin E

What it's for: Vitamin E is an antioxidant that helps protect cells, particularly those of the nervous system, from damage. There is some evidence to suggest that eating a diet high in vitamin E during pregnancy may protect your baby from developing asthma and other allergies.

Amount needed: Requirements for vitamin E depend on the amount of polyunsaturated fatty acids (PUFA) you consume. Individuals with higher PUFA intakes require more vitamin E, so there are no recommended levels for the general population. However, intakes around 4–5mg per day appear to be satisfactory for the majority of women who are pregnant or breastfeeding.

Where it's found: It is found in a wide variety of foods and getting enough isn't usually a problem for those eating a varied diet.

	Vitamin E (mg) per 100g	Vitamin E per portion
Spinach (raw)	1.7	1.4mg per 80g portion
Broccoli	1.2	1mg per 80g portion
Carrots	0.6	0.6mg per 80g portion
Tomatoes	1.2	1mg per tomato
Apples	0.6	0.6mg per medium apple
Almonds	24	7.2mg per 30g handful
Hazelnuts	25	7.5mg per 30g handful
Rapeseed oil	22	2.4mg per tablespoon
Olive oil	5	0.5mg per tablespoon

Source: Data taken from the UK Nutrient Databank © Crown copyright 2012

Calcium

What it's for: Calcium helps build strong bones and teeth. It also regulates muscle contraction and is needed for normal blood clotting.

Amount needed: Before and during pregnancy you need 700mg of calcium per day. This increases to 1,250mg per day for breastfeeding. To help your body absorb calcium, it's important to have enough vitamin D. Vegetarians who drink milk and have milk products such as cheese and yogurt every day usually consume plenty of calcium. However, research has shown that vegans have substantially lower intakes of calcium than other individuals. A large study, which included more than 1,000 vegans living in the UK, found that 76% of them had calcium intakes below the recommended 700mg. Far fewer meat-eaters (15%) and lacto-ovo-vegetarians (18%) had such low intakes. This same study, known as EPIC (European Prospective Investigation into Cancer and nutrition) found that the fracture rate was 30% higher for vegans than for meat-eaters.

Where it's found: Calcium is found in milk and dairy products and also in a variety of leafy green vegetables. Humans absorb about 30% of the calcium they consume, and how much you get from a particular meal depends on a variety of factors. Absorption is reduced in foods containing oxalic acid (including spinach, collard greens and rhubarb) and phytic acid (wholegrain cereals, beans and seeds) as these compounds bind to the calcium, so it carries on moving through the digestive tract and out. There was speculation that phosphate, which is found in fizzy drinks, also reduces calcium absorption, but recent research suggests that the link between fizzy drinks and lower bone mineral levels is due to people drinking them instead of milk.

The best sources of calcium for vegans include almonds, sesame seeds, tofu containing calcium chloride (E509), low-oxalic-acid leafy vegetables, and fortified foods. Almond butter may be better than whole almonds, as crushing the nuts makes the calcium more accessible, otherwise pieces of nut can pass through undigested. Likewise, tahini may be better than whole sesame seeds. Fortified foods can also make a huge difference to calcium intake, including milk alternatives and some bread. But remember to read the label, as products may look almost identical but one will have added calcium and not the other. If you usually drink rice milk or organic soya milk, check the label, as it probably doesn't have calcium added.

	Calcium (mg) per 100g	Calcium per portion
Milk	120	360mg per half-pint/300ml
Yogurt (plain)	162	202mg per small pot
Cheese	720	216mg per 30g portion
Fortified soya milk, hemp milk, oat milk or coconut milk	120	360mg per half-pint/300ml
Alpro soya desserts*	120	150mg per small pot
Burgen soya and linseed bread*	275	121mg per slice
Almonds	240	72mg per 30g handful
Almond butter	240	72mg per 3 teaspoons
Brazil nuts	170	51mg per 30g handful
Tofu	100-500	100-500mg per 100g portion
Sesame seeds/tahini	670	67mg per teaspoon

	Calcium (mg) per 100g	Calcium per portion
Broccoli	56	45mg per 80g portion
Curly kale	130	104mg per 80g portion
Chinese cabbage	54	43mg per 80g portion
Orange juice with added calcium (Tropicana)*	122	244mg per 200ml glass

*These figures are correct at the time of writing but manufacturers may change product ingredients, so it is best to check food labels.

Source: Data taken from various sources including the UK Nutrient Databank © Crown copyright 2012

Zinc

What it's for: Zinc is needed to make new cells and enzymes and to help wounds heal. The body also needs zinc to process the protein, carbohydrates and fats we eat.

Amount needed: During pregnancy you need 7mg of zinc per day. This increases to 13mg per day if you are breastfeeding exclusively, and 9.5mg a day once your baby is also having other food. Some studies have found that lacto-ovo-vegetarians have lower intakes of zinc than meat-eaters, but other studies have found similar levels. The EPIC study found that lacto-ovo-vegetarians had lower zinc intakes than meat-eaters and fish-eaters. Vegans had lower intakes still, but the average intake for all groups met the recommended level of 7mg per day. Meat is rich in zinc, but those who eat plenty of wholegrain foods also have a good intake. Vegetarians actually tend to absorb less zinc because of higher fibre and phytate intakes, but blood tests have found that lacto-ovo-vegetarians generally have adequate levels in their blood.

Where it's found: Zinc is found in milk, milk products and wholegrain cereal products. Although wheatgerm and bran are rich in zinc, little is absorbed due to high phytic acid levels.

	Zinc (mg) per 100g	Zinc per portion
Milk	0.4	1.2mg per half-pint/300ml
Cheddar	2.3	0.7mg per 30g portion
Wholemeal bread	1.6	1.3mg per two slices
Pine nuts	6.5	0.9mg per tablespoon
Nori seaweed (dried)	6.4	0.2mg per 2.5g sheet
Wholemeal pasta	1.2	2.4mg per 240g portion
Bran flakes	2.5	1mg per 40g bowl
Muesli	2.3	1.2mg per 50g bowl

Source: Data taken from the UK Nutrient Databank © Crown copyright 2012

Iodine

What it's for: Iodine is important for the development of the nervous system, particularly during the first three months of pregnancy. Babies of iodine-deficient women can have poor mental development. Iodine is also needed for the production of thyroid hormones. Deficiency is extremely rare in European countries, but women with marginal intakes can start to show signs of deficiency during pregnancy. The most obvious sign of deficiency is a goitre, which is a large swelling on the neck.

Amount needed: 140µg per day.

Where it's found: The main sources of iodine for lacto-ovo-vegetarians are milk and milk products. Research has shown that organic milk has around 40% of the level of iodine contained in conventional milk, reflecting the lower iodine intake of the cows. Therefore if you have organic milk, it's important to ensure you get enough iodine from other sources. Using salt with iodine added (iodised salt) is one way of increasing your intake, but obviously lots of salt isn't good for heart health.

Seaweed is an excellent source of iodine and is becoming increasingly easy to find. Dried seaweed is available in healthfood shops and many supermarkets, or if you know what you're doing, you can get it from the sea. You need to be careful about what type of seaweed you eat and how much you have, as some varieties contain incredibly high levels of iodine, so it is easy to have too much (see table). Very high intakes can interfere with thyroid function and it is not advisable to have more than about 300μg of iodine per day. The Vegan Society suggests that kombu is a good source of iodine, as it seems to have a fairly consistent iodine content. If you have a shaker in the kitchen containing 15g, this is sufficient for one person for a year (about 180μg per day). It may be easier to monitor if you have a smaller amount – say 3g for three months' supply (around 145μg per day).

	Iodine (μg) per 100g	Iodine per portion
Milk (conventional, not organic)	25–30	75–90μg per half-pint/ 300ml
Cheddar	39	11μg per 30g portion
Nori (dried seaweed)	1,470	36μg per 2.5g sheet
Wakame (dried seaweed)	16,830	168μg per 1g
Kombu or kelp (dried seaweed)	440,670	4,400μg per 1g

Source: Data taken from the UK Nutrient Databank © Crown copyright 2012

High intakes: Cases of vegetarians having excessively high intakes of iodine are occasionally reported. These are usually associated with high intakes of kelp but there is also a risk if several different sources of iodine are taken, for example iodised salt, seaweed and supplements. If you are getting iodine from several sources, it's important to monitor your intake.

Selenium

What it's for: Selenium is an antioxidant and therefore protects against cell damage. It also plays an important role in the immune system, thyroid hormone metabolism and reproduction. Research suggests that having a good intake of selenium during pregnancy may reduce the risk of your baby developing eczema and wheezing, which can be an early sign of asthma.

Amount needed: Women are advised to consume 60µg per day in pregnancy and 75µg per day while breastfeeding. Selenium intakes in the UK have fallen since the 1970s when we started eating more wheat from Europe and less from North America, where the soil is more selenium-rich. Average intakes are now below recommended levels for meat-eaters and vegetarians alike. Studies comparing selenium intakes and blood levels of selenium in lacto-ovo-vegetarians, vegans and meat-eaters have had mixed results, with some concluding that vegetarians' intakes are especially low but not others.

Where it's found: Selenium is not found in a wide range of foods. Brazil nuts are an excellent source and have been found to contain between 85 and 690µg per 100g, which is an incredibly wide range but reflects the levels found in different soils. If you have chocolate, or carob, coated brazils then you can have a treat but know you're getting something healthy too.

	Selenium (µg) per 100g	Selenium per portion
Brazil nuts (average)	254	76µg per 30g handful
Cashew nuts	29	9µg per 30g handful
Wholemeal bread	7	5µg per two slices
Eggs	11	13µg per two eggs
Lentils, cooked	40	32µg per 2 tablespoons
Kidney beans, cooked	6	5µg per 2 tablespoons

Source: Data taken from the UK Nutrient Databank © Crown copyright 2012

8 Omega 3 fatty acids – what's all the fuss about?

Most of us have heard of omega 3s. The term is often splashed across food and supplement labels, or bandied about in adverts, and there are whole books written about them. They appear to offer lots of health benefits, but the most common source is oily fish. So as a vegetarian do you really need them and if so where else can you get them?

The first thing to note is that there are several different kinds of omega 3s and not all of them provide the same benefits to your baby's health and development.

The science bit

Omega 3s are a type of fatty acid, the main component of fat. They are polyunsaturated and so are known as PUFAs (polyunsaturated fatty acids). There are two different categories, short-chain PUFAs and long-chain PUFAs (LCPUFAs). It is the long-chain ones that have been found to have particular benefits to babies' health.

The most important omega 3 fatty acids are:

- alpha linolenic acid (**ALA**): a short-chain omega 3 found in seeds and oils;
- docosahexaenoic acid (**DHA**): a long-chain omega 3 (LCPUFA) found mainly in oily fish, but also in small amounts in eggs and some algae;
- eicosapentaenoic acid (**EPA**): a long-chain omega 3 found in oily fish.

Food and supplement manufacturers often lump all omega 3s together, as if they had the same effects on health. Incidentally, short-chain omega 3s from vegetable oils are much cheaper to produce than long-chain omega 3s from fish or algae, so any confusion doesn't do profits any harm.

Alpha linolenic acid (ALA)

ALA is called an 'essential fatty acid'. This is because our bodies need it and it must be included in the diet. By contrast, our health wouldn't suffer if we didn't consume most of the other fatty acids found in food. There isn't an official recommendation for ALA intake but you need at least about 1g or 1,000mg per day.

Sources of short-chain omega 3 fatty acids are shown in the table for ALA.

	ALA (g) per 100g	ALA per portion
Flaxseeds (linseeds)	23	3.5g per tablespoon
Walnuts	9	2.5g per handful
Tofu	0.2	0.2g per 100g
Flaxseed oil	53	8g per tablespoon
Walnut oil	10	1.5g per tablespoon
Rapeseed oil	9	1.4g per tablespoon
Soya oil	7	1.1g per tablespoon

Source: Data taken from the U.S. Department of Agriculture, Agricultural Research Service, 2012. USDA National Nutrient Database for Standard Reference, Release 25. Nutrient Data Laboratory Home Page, www.ars.usda.gov/nutrientdata

Flaxseeds

Flaxseeds are a good source of ALA, but while you're pregnant you should avoid high intakes of whole or crushed flaxseeds because their husks contain lignins, which have a hormone-like effect. This makes them good for treating hot flushes during the menopause, but they may have undesirable effects during pregnancy. In animal studies, high intakes have been found to result in reduced litter size and birth weight.

You can avoid lignins by having flaxseed oil instead, since lignins are only found in the husk of flaxseeds. (But don't get 'high lignin flaxseed oil', which has lignins added to it.)

Docosahexaenoic acid (DHA)

Why you need DHA

DHA is vital for the development of your baby's brain, nervous system and the retina of the eye. Experts believe it's also required for other tissues, such as the heart. During pregnancy a baby accumulates roughly 10g of DHA, 6–7g of which is for brain development during the last trimester. A woman's DHA levels increase by about 50% during the first part of pregnancy in preparation for meeting her baby's needs later on.

The official advice

Pregnant and breastfeeding women require at least 200mg of DHA per day, according to a group of over 30 experts set up by the European Commission. The European Food Standards Agency (EFSA) advises that all adults consume a combined total of 250mg of DHA and EPA for their cardio-vascular health. In addition to this, women who are pregnant or breastfeeding should have an extra 100 to 200mg of DHA per day. Following this advice would mean your intake would be equivalent to eating one or two portions of oily fish a week, which is what the UK government recommends for pregnant women in general.

DHA in the diet

Many vegetarians consume no DHA at all, since it is found primarily in oily fish. Lacto-ovo-vegetarians can get small amounts of DHA by eating eggs or higher intakes if they eat eggs from chickens fed an omega 3-rich diet, such as Goldenlay (which have 150mg of LCPUFAs per egg). DHA is also found in some algae, and in the US more than 100 food products are now fortified with DHA from algal oil. This is starting to happen in the UK too, but at the moment the only widely available products containing algal oil are Quorn fishless fingers, which contain 29mg of LCPUFAs per finger. We are likely to see more foods fortified in this way in the future, but at the moment lacto-ovo-vegetarians in the UK are unlikely to meet recommendations from diet alone. For vegans it is even more difficult, as although some seaweeds contain very small amounts, getting it this way requires considerable expertise. Therefore taking supplements with DHA derived from algae is a good option.

Conversion

Your body can make DHA (a long-chain omega 3) from ALA (a short-chain omega 3). But this is not generally very effective and conversion rates vary among individuals. There is some speculation that the body becomes more efficient at turning ALA into DHA during pregnancy, but this has not been proved. When pregnant Dutch women were given ALA supplements, their blood DHA levels weren't found to increase and nor were their babies' levels. Another study, carried out in America, found that even when breastfeeding women took high doses of flaxseed oil (20g per day) it made no difference to the DHA levels in their milk. Experts generally believe you are unlikely to get enough long-chain omega 3s just by eating ALA-rich foods or taking supplements containing ALA.

Part of the problem is that high intakes of omega 6 fatty acids, which are found in sunflower oil, disrupt the conversion of ALA to DHA. This is a particular issue for vegetarians, who tend to have a high ratio of omega 6 to omega 3 fatty acids in their diets. However, this ratio can be lowered by replacing sunflower oil or corn oil with rapeseed oil or olive oil, and eating more ALA-rich foods, such as walnuts and flaxseeds (see table on page 126). Conversion of ALA to DHA is also more efficient if individuals are getting enough micro-nutrients, including iron, calcium, zinc and vitamin B_{12}.

Rapeseed oil
Rapeseed (canola) oil is a good general oil for cooking. As well as being lower in omega 6 fatty acids, it contains less saturated fat (7%) than butter (52%) or even olive oil (14%). It is also more stable than olive oil when heated, and it can be used in baking without affecting the flavour of cakes or other foods. Cold-pressed rapeseed oil is thought to be particularly beneficial.

DHA supplements

When you're pregnant

Since it is hard to get the recommended amount of DHA from your diet, you may want to take supplements. The evidence is not as strong as for folic acid supplements, but it is generally agreed that they are beneficial during pregnancy.

Research from several countries has shown that pregnant women who take DHA supplements have pregnancies that are 2-4 days longer on average and are less likely to give birth very prematurely (before 34 weeks). The babies of women on supplements have also been found to be heavier, 50-70g more on average. Being born too soon or too small can have serious health effects, although it is debatable whether a couple of days, or a couple of ounces, really makes much difference.

Scientists have also investigated how DHA supplements affect babies' health and development. Various studies have found that consuming higher levels of DHA during pregnancy and just after birth has beneficial effects on a baby's visual acuity, cognitive function, attention, maturity of sleep patterns and spontaneous motor activity. Different studies have looked at different features of development, so it is difficult to draw together the evidence and assess the overall impact. But higher levels of DHA certainly do seem to have a positive impact.

Another possible benefit of DHA is on allergy risk. It seems that taking supplements during pregnancy may help to protect babies against common food allergies, such as egg allergy, as well as reducing the risk of other allergic conditions, including eczema.

When you're breastfeeding

In the first few months of life, babies' brains continue to grow rapidly and accumulate DHA. If women don't consume any DHA themselves, their breast milk contains much less, though it still has some. The breast milk of vegan mothers who don't take DHA supplements has been found to have about a quarter the level of DHA found among meat-eaters. How this affects a baby isn't completely clear. Researchers have tried to see what difference it makes if breastfeeding mothers take DHA supplements. But trials involving mothers of full-term (rather than premature) babies haven't found any benefits to neurodevelopment (such as problem solving or motor skills). One study did find weak evidence of better language development at two years and of attention at five years when mothers took supplements.

Overall it remains debatable whether or not DHA supplements during breastfeeding provide clear benefits to a baby's development. It could be that any effects are only detectable when children are older and their cognitive function is more complex. Since there may be benefits, and there don't seem to be any adverse effects, supplementation is worth considering while you're breastfeeding.

Buying supplements

In the past, taking a DHA supplement meant taking a fish oil supplement, but in recent years supplements made from algal oil have become readily available and increasingly popular. This is partly because they are suitable for vegetarians, but also because they offer an alternative for anyone worried about contamination of fish with pollutants, and for those concerned about fish sustainability. Initially it wasn't known whether DHA from algae would be absorbed and used by the body in the same way as DHA from oily fish. However, research has shown that taking algal DHA supplements increases levels of DHA in the blood in the same way as eating salmon. It has also been found that breastfeeding women taking 200mg of DHA from algae have 75% higher DHA levels in their breast milk.

High-street pharmacy chains, such as Boots and Superdrug, don't seem to stock DHA supplements made from algae. However, some healthfood shops do and you can also get them online by searching for vegetarian DHA supplements. Several brands, including Opti 3, Deva and V-Pure, are approved by the Vegetarian Society and the Vegan Society. Each of these contains slightly different amounts of DHA and EPA, but they all seem like reasonable choices based on the official recommendations above. No doubt there are also other brands that would fit the bill. It is best not to take supplements containing more than 1g (1,000mg) of DHA or 2.7g of long-chain omega 3s per day. Research studies have used this amount without any adverse effects, but the effects of taking higher doses are unknown.

Some people take spirulina, which is a type of algae that can be bought in powder or tablet form. It is known to be rich in DHA, as well as containing vitamins and minerals. However, it has not been tested for safety during pregnancy, and the official advice from the National Institutes of Health (NIH) in the US is that it is best avoided in pregnancy and breastfeeding, to be on the safe side.

9 Should I take supplements?

While there is some debate about whether you need omega 3 supplements (page 129), there is clear evidence that certain other supplements are beneficial. Those containing folic acid and vitamin D are recommended for all pregnant women, irrespective of their diet. Other supplements, such as iron tablets, should only be taken during pregnancy if blood tests show they are needed. Manufacturers offer a whole range of other supplements they claim are essential for all mums-to-be. Some of these might be worth taking, but you may not need them. You should think about your own diet and look at the evidence before deciding what to do.

Folic acid and vitamin D

The government advises all pregnant women to take:

- 400µg of folic acid daily before conception and for the first 12 weeks of pregnancy;
- 10µg of vitamin D daily for the entire course of pregnancy and while breastfeeding.

Folic acid supplements

There is strong evidence that folic acid supplements reduce the risk of having a baby with a neural tube defect (NTD) such as spina bifida or anencephaly. In fact, trials with folic acid had to be stopped early because the benefits were so clear that it was unethical to continue giving some women a placebo.

Ideally you should start taking folic acid supplements before you become pregnant, but otherwise begin as soon as possible and continue until week 12 of pregnancy. It's safe to continue taking folic acid beyond 12 weeks, but there is generally no need if you are eating well. Supplements are available from chemists and most supermarkets quite cheaply, or you may be eligible to get them free (see page 140).

Supplements containing 400µg of folic acid (sometimes written as 0.4mg, 400mcg or 400 micrograms) are recommended for most women. However, some may benefit from even higher doses, of up to 5mg (5,000µg). If you have had a previous pregnancy affected by an NTD, or if you or your partner has a family history of NTDs, or if you are diabetic, then ask your doctor about taking a higher dose of folic acid. Unless you have been advised to take more than the recommended 400µg per day, it is best not to take more than 1,000µg (1mg) per day.

Vitamin B$_6$ supplements

There is a small amount of evidence suggesting that vitamin B$_6$ supplements can relieve nausea and vomiting in pregnancy in some women. If you're feeling dreadful you may be willing to try anything, but they should be treated with caution. The FSA advises against taking more than 10mg of supplemental vitamin B$_6$ per day. Taking very large doses

(200mg a day) is associated with nerve damage and loss of feeling in the hands and feet, which may be irreversible. A report by NICE suggests that taking smaller doses, up to 40mg a day, should be considered. If you want to try supplements, it is best to talk to your doctor before starting.

Research in Thailand found that vitamin B_6 supplements weren't as effective as either ginger or acupressure at relieving nausea and vomiting, so you may like to try some wristbands or ginger first.

Vitamin B_{12} supplements

If you don't have eggs, dairy foods or foods fortified with vitamin B_{12} (see page 109) every day then you need to take a supplement. If you're relying on fortified foods then try to work out roughly how much vitamin B_{12} you are having each day. If you think that some days you might not get as much as recommended, then it is best to take a supplement. Taking a multivitamin and mineral supplement that includes it is probably easiest.

Vitamin D supplements

The government advises women to take supplements containing 10μg (10mcg, 10 micrograms, 400 international units, 400i.u.) of vitamin D throughout pregnancy and while breastfeeding. Low levels of vitamin D during pregnancy can be detrimental to both mother and baby and can result in weak bones and infantile seizures (see page 113).

About a third of young women have low levels of vitamin D in their blood. Those most at risk are women who don't get much sunlight, women of South Asian, African, Caribbean or

Middle Eastern descent, women who are obese, and women who have recently been pregnant. Vegetarians have also been found to have lower levels than others. Women who have low levels of vitamin D when they become pregnant don't have adequate stores to draw on.

Blood tests for vitamin D status aren't routinely carried out, so you're unlikely to know whether you are among the one in three with low levels. Therefore supplements really are a good idea. Most supplements contain vitamin D3 from sheep's wool (see page 114), but D2 supplements are also available. Evidence suggests that D2 isn't as good when given as a single large dose, but it may not make a difference when taken as a daily supplement. The other option is to take a D3 supplement suitable for vegans, which may be derived from lichen. Unfortunately this is likely to be more expensive and it will be more difficult to get a supplement containing just the recommended 10µg per day.

It is important not to take too much vitamin D, as very high intakes can lead to more calcium being absorbed than the body is able to excrete, resulting in kidney damage. In the long term it can also result in weak bones, as calcium is drawn out of them. Taking supplements containing more than about 25µg (1,000i.u.) of vitamin D is not advisable. Don't worry about overdosing through too much sunlight, as this isn't possible, but choose your vitamin D supplement carefully.

Calcium supplements

If you don't have milk, milk products or a milk-alternative with added calcium, you are unlikely to be getting enough calcium for pregnancy or breastfeeding and should take a calcium supplement. Most multivitamin and mineral supplements don't contain 100% of the recommended calcium intake, partly because you need so much of it and this would make the tablets quite large. Besides, if a single tablet did include all the 700mg needed for pregnancy, your body wouldn't be able to process it. The percentage of calcium absorbed from a supplement is reduced at higher doses. So, if you are taking 1,000mg of calcium a day, it is better to have it as two 500mg tablets at different times of the day, rather than all at once.

Calcium supplements are usually either calcium carbonate or calcium citrate. Side-effects, including wind, bloating and constipation, are reported more often with calcium carbonate, so if you are having these problems you might want to switch. Spreading your supplements through the day and having them with meals may also help relieve side-effects. If you suffer from digestive problems and take an antacid, check whether it contains calcium carbonate as this will add to your calcium intake.

Iron supplements

If blood tests show you are anaemic, then you need to take iron supplements (see page 99). Otherwise it is fine to have iron if it is included in a pregnancy multivitamin and mineral supplement, but taking a high-dose iron supplement could be detrimental. If you are taking iron supplements and a multivitamin and mineral supplement, it is best to take them at different times of the day, as iron competes for absorption with other minerals, such as zinc.

Fluoride supplements

These are not recommended. There is some evidence that taking fluoride supplements during pregnancy reduces the risk of your child developing tooth decay. However, this research is controversial, as other studies have found no benefit. There is also some suggestion, although it has not been researched properly, that taking fluoride supplements in pregnancy could adversely affect foetal brain development.

Omega 3 supplements

There are several different types of omega 3 supplements available and as we've seen they don't all offer the same health benefits (page 125). If you want to take an omega 3 supplement, it's important to read the small print and see if it contains DHA, which appears to be beneficial, or ALA, which has not been found to have the same effects.

Supplements containing cod liver oil, or other fish liver oils, are high in beneficial omega 3s. However, they are not suitable for pregnancy, because they contain high levels of vitamin A, which could harm your baby.

Multivitamin and mineral supplements

If you think you might not be getting the recommended amounts of different nutrients then a multivitamin and mineral supplement is a good idea. A general supplement for pregnancy and breastfeeding provides a good safeguard for anyone with a limited diet.

It is not advisable to take a multivitamin and mineral supplement that is not specifically for pregnancy, as it may not contain the right balance of nutrients. For example, it might have too much vitamin A or not enough folic acid. If you compare the labels on the different pregnancy brands, you'll find they do vary. Most contain folic acid and vitamin D, which the government recommends for all pregnant women. They also tend to include iron, zinc and vitamin B_{12}. Some contain calcium, iodine and selenium, but other popular brands don't. Unless you're confident that you're getting adequate amounts of these nutrients, look for a supplement that includes them.

It is theoretically possible to take a variety of supplements containing individual nutrients. However, it is very difficult to get the right amount of each nutrient and not have too much of any. More is not necessarily better when it comes to nutrients, and the effect of having large doses of some of them is unknown. A study using high doses of vitamins C and E found that the desired effect of preventing pre-eclampsia wasn't achieved, but there was an increased number of babies with low birth weights – so caution is important. Another issue is that certain nutrients work together, for example vitamin D helps calcium absorption, so it's a good idea to have these nutrients together. Other nutrients, such as iron and zinc, compete for absorption, so taking too much of one will reduce absorption of the other.

If you are a vegan and are not happy taking vitamin D3 from sheep's wool, then you will have to shop around very carefully to see if you can find a suitable supplement, as most multivitamins use this type of vitamin D.

If you think your diet is probably sufficient, you may be wondering whether or not to take a multivitamin and mineral supplement. Several studies have looked at the effect of supplements in well-nourished women, with mixed results. On balance, the evidence suggests that they are either beneficial or have no effect. It's difficult to determine the impact of supplements, because the women who take them are less likely to drink alcohol or smoke and more likely to eat well and exercise. It could be that some of the benefits associated with supplements are due to these factors rather than to the supplements themselves.

It is important to remember that a multivitamin and mineral supplement is not a substitute for a good diet. For one thing, real fruits and vegetables contain beneficial phytochemicals, such as lycopene in tomatoes and anthocyanins in blackberries and aubergines, which are not found in most supplements. So, if you take a supplement, you should still try to eat as well as possible. It is best to take any supplements during or after a meal in order to maximise nutrient absorption.

Supplements for diabetic mums-to-be
If you have diabetes, then taking a multivitamin and mineral supplement is probably a good idea, as well as a higher dose of folic acid. A study in the US found that, although diabetic women generally have an increased risk of having a baby with a birth defect such as hydrocephalus or a heart defect, those taking multivitamins before and during pregnancy have no greater risk than non-diabetic women.

Healthy Start

If you are on a low income, you may be eligible for free supplements through the Healthy Start scheme. The scheme helps pregnant women and mothers of young children who are on low income or receiving certain benefits. In addition, all pregnant women under the age of 18 qualify. Women who are eligible receive free supplements (containing folic acid and vitamins C and D) and vouchers for free fruit, vegetables and milk. The vitamin D in the supplements is D3, which is extracted from the wool of living sheep. They can also be bought from some pharmacies or online. To find out more about Healthy Start see Resources, or ask your doctor, midwife or health visitor.

10 Common complaints and how to deal with them

It would be wonderful if every woman could spend her pregnancy feeling radiant with health and vitality. However, most experience some kind of problem, even if it's just mild morning sickness or heartburn. Looking after yourself with regular meals, fresh air, rest and sleep are really important during pregnancy and can make a big difference to both your physical and your emotional well-being.

Some of the common problems of pregnancy can be helped by making changes to the foods you eat, or the way you eat them. This is true for problems with an obvious dietary link such as constipation, but also when it comes to certain other issues, including restless legs and sleep problems.

Morning sickness

If you're suffering from morning sickness, you're in good company: about three-quarters of women experience some feelings of nausea during pregnancy. The intensity of the symptoms can vary - about 30% of women are affected by severe nausea and vomiting. Despite being referred to as 'morning sickness', it can occur at any time of day. Some women find it gets worse if they are feeling tired, stressed or hungry. It can also be triggered by certain odours, such as cooking smells or strong aftershave. Generally symptoms are worst at around 9-10 weeks and disappear by around the fourteenth week of pregnancy. By the time women reach the third month of pregnancy, 90% find their symptoms have disappeared.

The exact cause of morning sickness isn't known, but it's thought to be related to increasing oestrogen levels and a sudden rise in human chorionic gonadotropin (hCG) levels in early pregnancy. This hormone, hCG, is the same one that gives you a positive pregnancy test. Women carrying twins are more likely to suffer from morning sickness, as they have higher levels of hCG in early pregnancy.

You may worry that your baby is suffering too. However, feeling sick is actually a sign that your hormone levels are changing as they should, and although you feel awful, your baby is very unlikely to be affected. Research shows that mothers who suffer from morning sickness are just as likely to have healthy babies as those who don't. Even if you're feeling so sick that you can't bear to eat a healthy meal, try not to worry. If you're not eating very much or not managing to keep much down, your baby will simply draw on your nutrient stores. Try eating small snacks throughout the day to help keep your energy levels up, and make these as healthy as possible, but if you can't face anything apart from plain crackers, salty crisps or sour sweets, then don't worry. These are better than nothing. Do what you can to relieve the symptoms and when you are feeling a bit better, try to eat more healthily.

Unfortunately, the time when morning sickness is likely to be at its worst is probably before you have told other people that you're pregnant. You may also be feeling especially emotional and still getting used to the idea of having a baby. This can be particularly difficult at work or if friends and family are expecting you to be your normal self.

There is no single treatment that works for all women, but different strategies can be helpful. You could try the following:

- Eat little and often. By eating small, carbohydrate-rich meals or snacks every couple of hours, you can stop your blood sugar levels dropping too low, which is often what makes women feel worse.

- Eat some dry crackers or ginger biscuits in bed before you get up in the morning.

- Avoid foods that trigger nausea, such as fatty or spicy dishes, or foods with a strong odour. It may be better to eat certain foods cold or, if you can, get someone else to do the cooking until you're feeling better. You could also stick to simple foods that don't have a strong odour, such as bread or baked potatoes.

- Avoid any other triggers. Some women find the smell of petrol, perfume or certain shops sets them off, or that travelling by bus or in the back of the car makes them feel sick.

- Vitamin B_6 supplements help some women suffering from morning sickness (see page 134).

- Have plenty of fluids to avoid dehydration, which can increase your feeling of nausea and also cause headaches. It may be better to sip water or other drinks throughout the day rather than having a large drink in one go, which can make vomiting more likely. It may also help if you avoid very cold drinks or those that taste sweet.

- Have ginger in any form possible. It's a traditional remedy and it really does seem to help. Several trials have been conducted in Australia and Thailand in recent years to test its effectiveness. These have found that taking 1g of ginger a day (or an equivalent amount in a capsule or syrup) is effective in reducing feelings of nausea and episodes of vomiting in the majority of women.

- Get more fresh air.
- Find something to distract you, even if it's just watching television or calling a friend.
- Rest and sleep as much as possible, as tiredness makes symptoms worse.
- Get some seasickness wristbands from a chemist. These act on the acupressure point for nausea. Some trials, though not all, have found them to be effective. You can also try stimulating the acupressure point yourself.
- Avoid clothes that are uncomfortable around your waist such as tights or anything with a tight waistband.
- Sip cider vinegar in water with meals or throughout the day. Put a few drops or a teaspoonful into a glass of cold or warm water. A teaspoon of honey can be added to make it taste better. There is no scientific evidence regarding whether or not it works, but there is no harm in trying. This remedy is more popular in the USA and some enthusiasts believe only unpasteurised cider vinegar is effective. However, this is not readily available in the UK and is best avoided because of the risk of food poisoning.
- Complementary therapies are helpful for some women. You can try acupuncture, a variety of homeopathic remedies or aromatherapy, including ginger, grapefruit, lavender or peppermint oil.

How to eat ginger
- Grate it into a stir-fry.
- Make a soup such as carrot and ginger, pumpkin and ginger or any veg you fancy.

- Have ginger biscuits or ginger cake.
- Eat crystallised ginger (candied ginger) as it is, or use it in baking or in tea.
- Have toast with ginger marmalade for breakfast.
- Buy non-alcoholic ginger beer or ginger ale. Check 'ginger extract' is listed as an ingredient, otherwise it may have ginger flavouring, which probably won't be effective.
- Make tea with grated ginger and boiled water. Try adding honey and lemon too.
- Get ginger chews, boiled sweets or chewing gum. Most healthfood shops sell a variety of products containing ginger.

A small number of women, around 1%, suffer from such severe vomiting during pregnancy (hyperemesis gravidarum) that they need to go into hospital. An article in the journal *Obstetrics and Gynecology* in 2011 questioned whether GPs in the UK should take the condition more seriously, as it is thought that better advice or treatment early on could avoid the need for hospitalisation. In the USA and Canada, severe morning sickness is treated with antihistamines and pyridoxine (vitamin B_6), but in the UK, GPs don't usually prescribe any drug treatment. If you've tried everything suggested here without success, then talk to your doctor about the options.

Warning - Calabash chalk, bentonite clay and Zam Zam water
Calabash chalk (also known as Calabar stone, La Craie, Argile, Nzu and Mabele) is a traditional West African remedy for morning sickness. It is sometimes imported to the UK, but the FSA has warned women not to take it because it has

▶

been found to contain high levels of lead, which could harm your baby's developing nervous system.

Another suggested remedy, bentonite clay, should also be avoided, as the FSA has found that it, and other clay-based drinks, contain high levels of lead and arsenic. It is usually drunk with water and is readily available on the Internet. It is sold on the basis that it detoxifies the liver of chemicals that cause morning sickness. Such claims are completely unsubstantiated.

Zam Zam water, which comes from Saudi Arabia and is sacred to Muslims, is believed to have many benefits, including relieving morning sickness and making pregnancy and labour easier. However, tests carried out on water labelled as Zam Zam water in the UK, including samples brought into the country for personal use, identified arsenic levels almost three times the legal limit. Because of associations between arsenic and increased risk of several types of cancer, this too should be avoided in pregnancy.

Heartburn

While morning sickness tends to strike at the beginning of pregnancy, heartburn is more likely to be a problem in the last three months. The main symptom is a burning sensation in the chest, caused by acids going back up the oesophagus (food pipe) from the stomach. A muscle valve usually prevents this from happening, but during pregnancy hormonal changes cause muscle relaxation and the valve becomes less effective.

Heartburn can be particularly bad after a large meal or during activities that involve bending down, such as cleaning the floor or even just picking something up. The pressure of the growing baby on the stomach can make heartburn worse as pregnancy progresses. This is particularly true for those expecting twins, as the uterus is inevitably larger and therefore presses more on the stomach. In the last weeks of pregnancy, your baby's head may move down into your pelvis in preparation for the birth. The head is then said to be 'engaged'. This usually reduces the pressure on the mother's stomach and the symptoms of heartburn are often reduced. The good news is that when the baby is delivered, heartburn generally disappears almost instantly.

There are several things you can do to ease the symptoms of heartburn:

- Wear loose-fitting clothes to reduce extra pressure on your stomach.
- Avoid becoming too full, by eating little and often instead of having large meals. Also, don't drink too much at mealtimes so that your stomach doesn't become so full.
- Try to identify trigger foods and avoid them, especially in the evening. Common culprits include spicy food, citrus fruits, rich and fatty foods, tea and coffee, and bananas.
- When you eat, sit upright instead of slouching, and try not to rush.
- Try staying upright for a while after meals and avoid eating for a couple of hours before going to bed.
- When you go to bed, prop yourself up with several pillows.
- Milk is good for neutralising the stomach acid and easing symptoms, so try drinking a small glass before bed or have some ready to sip during the night.
- Homeopathy, aromatherapy and yoga may all help.

If you suffer from severe heartburn then talk to your doctor or midwife. They will be able to prescribe a suitable antacid or anti-reflux medicine. Not all treatments are suitable for pregnancy, so before taking anything it is best to check with your doctor, your midwife or a pharmacist.

Excessive thirst

Many women feel more thirsty than usual during pregnancy. This is quite normal, as extra fluids are needed to allow your blood volume to increase and to produce and constantly replace the amniotic fluid your baby is swimming in. Some women also feel warmer than usual and lose water due to hot sweats, which further increases fluid needs. If your wee is dark yellow, this is a sign of dehydration and means you need to drink more. It may be due to severe morning sickness or it may be something simple, such as giving up coffee and not replacing it with other fluids. It's important to make sure you have at least eight glasses of fluid a day.

A small number of women experience such a raging thirst that they end up having to carry around litre bottles of water at all times. Generally this is nothing to worry about, although it is worth talking to your doctor or midwife about it. If you are weeing more than usual as well as feeling very thirsty, it can be a sign of gestational diabetes and your doctor or midwife can check if this is the case.

Constipation

Constipation isn't as common among vegetarians as among meat-eaters, and vegans tend to have less of a problem than lacto-ovo-vegetarians, as they usually have a higher fibre intake. However, constipation is more common for everyone during pregnancy because of hormonal changes. Increasing progesterone levels cause all the muscles in your body, including intestinal muscles, to relax, so food moves through your intestines more slowly. This helps your body absorb more nutrients from the food, but it can also lead to constipation. In addition, the pressure of your baby on your bowels can make going to the toilet more difficult. Iron supplements can also make matters worse. However, making a few adjustments to your diet and being as active as possible can go a long way towards easing the problem.

To treat constipation, try the following:

- Eat plenty of fibre-rich foods such as wholemeal bread, wholegrain breakfast cereal, pulses and lots of fruit and vegetables.

- Have some prunes or prune juice. This is an age-old remedy that really works. The laxative effect cannot be explained just by fibre – prunes contain similar amounts to other dried fruit, and prune juice has none at all, as it is filtered before bottling. It is more likely to be down to the high levels of sorbitol in prunes. This is a type of sugar that is absorbed very slowly and passes into the large intestine like fibre. Prunes also contain large amounts of phenolic compounds, which also have a natural laxative effect.

- Drink plenty of water and other fluids. Along with dietary fibre, water helps to make stools softer and bulkier, which means they are easier to pass.

- Take some gentle exercise, such as walking, swimming or yoga.

- When you go to the toilet, relax and take your time.

- Switch iron supplements if necessary (see page 99).

Ban bran

Sprinkling bran onto cereal or other foods may help relieve constipation but it isn't a good idea. Bran comes from the outer layer of cereal grains, such as wheat or rice, and it contains lots of fibre. The problem is that it reduces the absorption of important vitamins and minerals, including iron and zinc. It is much better to eat fibre-rich foods such as wholemeal bread, pulses, vegetables and fruit, as these contain higher levels of essential nutrients.

If you still have constipation, talk to your midwife or doctor; they may prescribe laxatives that are safe to take during pregnancy. Not all laxatives are suitable.

Wind and bloating

As well as being prone to constipation, pregnant women also experience more wind, bloating and general digestive discomfort. Food spends longer in the intestines so that more nutrients can be absorbed, but this also means that it has more time to ferment and produce gas or wind.

To relieve the symptoms of wind, bloating and general discomfort, try the following:

- Avoid foods that are particular triggers. Different foods seem to affect different people, but beans, cabbage and onions are common culprits. To prevent your diet becoming too limited, you could have individual trigger foods on different days, but avoid having several at the same time.
- Don't eat large meals.
- Try to relax and sit up tall at mealtimes.
- When you eat, chew properly, and avoid gulping air by eating slowly and not talking too much at the same time.
- Avoid swallowing air when you drink by using a cup or glass rather than drinking from a bottle or through a straw.
- Avoid fizzy drinks.
- Take gentle exercise such as yoga or walking to help keep your digestive system working efficiently.

If you are feeling pain rather than discomfort, talk to your doctor or midwife as soon as possible.

Haemorrhoids (piles)

Piles or haemorrhoids are swollen veins around the rectum and anus (back passage). If you have piles you can usually feel them as lumps. They can feel itchy or cause pain and aching. When you go to the toilet they can feel particularly uncomfortable or painful, and you may notice some blood on the toilet paper when you wipe your bottom.

Some women develop piles for the first time during pregnancy; others find existing piles may get worse. Piles are exacerbated by straining when you go to the toilet and by constipation. Vegetarians tend to suffer from piles less often than meat-eaters because they eat more foods of plant origin and have a higher fibre intake.

To treat piles:

- Follow the advice for constipation (page 151).
- Try not to strain when you go to the toilet.
- Use moist toilet wipes rather than toilet paper.
- If the piles stick out, push them gently back inside.
- Avoid standing up for long periods.

You can talk to your midwife, doctor or pharmacist about a suitable cream or ointment. This may help relieve the itching and inflammation but will not address the cause.

Generally piles become much better after your baby is born. Sometimes they can become worse - particularly if it is a difficult vaginal delivery. However, even then, they should improve as you recover from the birth.

Diarrhoea

Although diarrhoea is a much less common complaint than constipation during pregnancy, some women do find it a problem. There is nothing to worry about unless the diarrhoea is severe and continues for more than a few days. If that is the case, you should see your GP for further tests, such as a stool culture, to rule out salmonella and other infections.

Like so many pregnancy problems, diarrhoea can be caused by changing hormone levels. Though it can be unpleasant, it is not a problem in itself. However, it can cause dehydration. So, if you have diarrhoea, it is important to drink plenty of water or take a rehydration powder, which is available from a pharmacy. Taking a probiotic yogurt or drink may also help.

If you get diarrhoea towards the end of pregnancy, it can be one of the signs that your hormone levels are changing and your body is preparing for labour. It may be that labour is imminent, or mild diarrhoea may continue for several days before you go into labour.

Dizziness and fainting

Half to three-quarters of pregnant women experience dizziness at some time. You may find that you feel light-headed when you get out of bed in the morning or if you get up from a chair too quickly. Standing still for long periods might also make you feel light-headed.

There are several possible causes:

- low blood sugar levels due to not eating enough;
- low blood pressure – this is common in early pregnancy as progesterone causes the walls of the blood vessels to relax;

- low iron levels or anaemia;
- getting too hot.

Whatever the cause, the first thing to do is make sure you sit down, so that you don't fall down. It may help if you lie down on your left side or sit with your head between your knees, as this increases blood flow to your brain. When the immediate dizziness passes, it shouldn't be too difficult to work out if you need to eat or cool down and then remedy the problem. Your midwife should be able to tell you if you have low iron levels from the results of your blood tests, and if this is the case the problem can be treated with iron supplements (see page 99). Your midwife should also be able to tell you if you have low blood pressure, and if this is the case you just need to be more careful about getting up slowly and sitting down if you start to feel dizzy.

If you have actually fainted, it's best to see your doctor to make sure everything is okay. You should also do this if you experience other problems too, such as a headache, pelvic pain or blurred vision.

Restless legs

Restless Leg Syndrome (RLS) involves a strong urge to move the legs and also sometimes the arms. Women generally find symptoms are worse when they settle down for a much-needed rest, particularly at night. RLS can occur at any stage of life but is two to three times more likely during pregnancy, particularly in the last trimester. It is estimated that between 10% and 25% of women are affected at some stage of pregnancy. Symptoms usually disappear after the baby is born.

It is not clear what causes RLS, but people who suffer from it have been found to have lower levels of dopamine in a region of the brain known as the substantia niagra. Iron is important in the production of dopamine, and low iron levels may be part of the problem. Certainly RLS appears to be more common in pregnant women with low iron levels, and symptoms tend to improve when iron supplements are given. In addition, folic acid supplements have been found to help alleviate symptoms, although the reason for this is less clear. Some people find that particular foods or drinks act as a trigger, for example coffee or sugary foods.

To help relieve restless legs, try the following:

- Take some exercise every day, but avoid exercising vigorously just before bed.
- Stretch your legs and massage them before you settle down for the night.
- Take a warm bath before bed.
- Avoid refined sugars and instead eat more low-GI foods.
- Avoid caffeine completely, as this may have some effect.
- If your iron levels are low, take iron supplements. You can also try folic acid supplements.
- Try stretching, bending and rubbing your legs or walking around the room when symptoms occur.

Sleep problems and tiredness

Sleep problems are common in pregnancy, as it can be difficult to find a comfortable position as your bump grows. It can also be difficult to get a good night's sleep if you're suffering from nausea or heartburn or find yourself having to get up for a wee. Worrying, or even just thinking, about your baby and the future may also keep you awake.

Eight hours of sound sleep may not be possible for some time (maybe for years), but there are plenty of things you can do to improve the quality of your sleep and help you feel refreshed when you get up in the morning:

- Use extra pillows and cushions to make yourself more comfortable. Using a foam wedge under your bump or a V- or U-shaped cushion may help.

- Avoid exercise late in the evening as this can interfere with sleep patterns. Regular exercise will help you to sleep more soundly but it is better to do this earlier in the day.

- Have a bedtime routine that includes quiet time and a warm bath before bed. Once you're in bed there shouldn't be any electronic devices such as laptops or smartphones; some quiet music or a book is much better. You should also try to get to bed at about the same time every night and avoid napping on the sofa beforehand.

- Avoid having any caffeine in the afternoon and evening.

- Don't have a large meal just before bed, as this can lead to indigestion and heartburn (see page 148). Instead have regular meals, including breakfast, lunch and an early evening meal, then maybe a small snack later on.

- Drink plenty of fluids during the day but avoid having too much to drink in the evening.

- Have a warm milky drink in the evening.

You're bound to feel tired if you haven't slept well, but having a lack of energy and generally feeling lethargic can have other causes, including anaemia and gestational diabetes, so talk to your doctor or midwife about it. In early pregnancy tiredness can be a particular problem, as hormone levels are altered, your body is starting to change and you're probably still trying to do everything you would normally do. The obvious remedy is to slow down and look after yourself by eating and sleeping well.

Gestational diabetes

This is a temporary form of diabetes that affects about 5% of pregnant women. It develops when hormones from the placenta interfere with insulin, the hormone that regulates blood sugar levels. As a result, the level of glucose or sugar in your blood can rise and dip steeply. You are more likely to develop gestational diabetes mellitus (GDM) if you have a family history of diabetes, have had a very large baby before, have a BMI over 30, or are of South Asian, black Caribbean or Middle Eastern origin.

Gestational diabetes is usually detected at 24-28 weeks of pregnancy. The first sign is likely to be glucose in your urine. A single positive test is not generally seen as a cause for concern. But if glucose is found on several occasions, or if you are at high risk of GDM, you may be given an oral glucose tolerance test (OGTT or GTT). This involves having a blood test before breakfast and another two hours later after having a glucose drink.

Women who develop the condition, like those who have diabetes before pregnancy, are likely to have bigger-than-average babies. This is because the baby receives more glucose, and therefore more calories, than normal. This in turn increases the likelihood of problems during delivery, including the need for a caesarean. If blood sugar levels aren't controlled, it can also affect the development of a baby's heart and lungs and increase their chances of developing obesity and diabetes in later life. However, if the condition is controlled carefully, it should not harm you or your baby.

To combat the effects of gestational diabetes, you need to keep your blood sugar levels as stable as possible so that the baby doesn't receive extra glucose. This can be done by changing what you eat and exercising more, which isn't always easy. The most important thing is to avoid high-sugar foods and drinks, including fruit juices, and to have low-GI carbohydrates whenever possible (see page 36). Some people may need extra insulin. If you have gestational diabetes, you will be given more frequent antenatal appointments to check that you and your baby are both well. You should also receive advice about what to eat and how to monitor your blood glucose levels.

After the birth, the condition usually goes away completely. Both you and your baby will have your blood glucose levels checked after delivery. Unfortunately, having GDM during one pregnancy increases the chances of developing it in future pregnancies, particularly if you are overweight. Also, according to Diabetes UK, women with GDM have a 30% chance of developing Type 2 diabetes at some time during their life, compared to a 10% chance in the general population.

Pre-eclampsia

This is a potentially serious pregnancy disorder characterised by high blood pressure, swelling due to fluid retention and protein in the urine. Other symptoms may include headaches and blurred vision. An estimated one in 20 pregnancies is affected. You are more likely to develop pre-eclampsia if you are severely overweight, aged over 40 or expecting more than one baby, or if any of your close relatives has had it.

Mild cases of pre-eclampsia have no significant effect on pregnancy, but if the condition isn't treated, it can progress to a more serious condition called eclampsia. Severe cases can result in convulsions and, very occasionally, death. However, drugs can usually be given to treat the symptoms of pre-eclampsia and, if necessary, the baby will be delivered early.

A good diet appears to reduce the risk of pre-eclampsia. When the medical records of 775 mothers living in a vegan community in Tennessee were examined, only one case of pre-eclampsia was found (0.1%). This is much lower than expected and is probably related to the women's healthy balanced diet, multivitamin and mineral supplement intake, and generally healthy lifestyle. Research has also shown that pre-eclampsia is less common in women with higher intakes of antioxidants. Having a healthy diet, rich in vitamins C and E, appears to be particularly important, although vitamin C and E supplements do not have the same effect (see page 139). Multivitamin and mineral supplements might, however, help prevent pre-eclampsia, according to another study. It has also been found that calcium supplements may help protect against pre-eclampsia for women who have low intakes of calcium. This is another good reason to make sure you get enough calcium.

Research has also looked at whether garlic and chocolate might reduce the incidence of pre-eclampsia. It is thought that garlic may help by lowering blood pressure, but findings have been inconclusive. In 2010, the media reported that eating chocolate halved the risk of premature birth, because it prevented pre-eclampsia. However, these claims weren't backed up by the evidence. It does seem plausible that chocolate might reduce the risk of pre-eclampsia, as studies in the past have shown dark chocolate may reduce the risk of heart disease, possibly by lowering blood pressure. A study from the USA found that women who ate chocolate at least once a week during pregnancy reduced their risk of pre-eclampsia by 50%. This sounds pretty convincing but it may be a case of 'reverse causality' - maybe women with pre-eclampsia eat less chocolate because of their diagnosis, rather than women who eat less chocolate getting pre-eclampsia more often. Cause and effect couldn't be differentiated in the study.

Foods to kick-start labour – or not

If your due date comes and goes and nothing seems to be happening, it can be very frustrating, particularly if family and friends start calling to see what's happening. There are many myths and old wives' tales about what you can do to kick-start labour – some of the ideas are more pleasant than others. When it comes to diet, there are several suggestions:

- raspberry leaf;
- evening primrose;
- pineapple;
- curry.

Raspberry leaf is thought to be a uterine stimulant which helps strengthen the muscles of the womb, so that contractions are more effective and labour is easier. Several trials have been carried out, including an Australian study in which women were given either two raspberry leaf supplements (1.2g each) or two placebo tablets a day from 32 weeks of pregnancy. It was found that the second stage of labour (pushing the baby out) was 10 minutes shorter in the group who took raspberry leaf. They also had a lower rate of forceps delivery (19% versus 30%). However, they didn't go into labour any sooner.

Although raspberry leaf doesn't seem to bring on labour, the general advice is not to take it until you are at least 32 weeks' pregnant. You should also talk to your midwife first as it isn't suitable for everyone and probably isn't a good idea if you've previously had quite a quick labour, you're expecting twins or you've had problems such as high blood pressure or vaginal bleeding. If you do decide to give it a try, you can either drink raspberry leaf tea or, if you don't like the taste, take raspberry leaf tablets or capsules.

Some women take evening primrose supplements, or use them vaginally, to kick-start labour. Although some people swear by them, because they took them and went into labour, there is no objective evidence that they are more effective than just waiting. The National Institute of Health in the US advises pregnant women not to take evening primrose oil because, although evidence is inconclusive, it could possibly increase the risk of complications.

Fresh pineapple could theoretically help, as it contains an enzyme called bromelain, which breaks down proteins. In a highly concentrated form, bromelain is used to treat inflammation. Taking bromelain tablets or capsules during pregnancy is not recommended, however, as it may cause abnormal bleeding. However, some alternative therapists may recommend them at the end of pregnancy to help soften and dilate the cervix, although there is no evidence that this is effective. To get enough bromelain from fresh pineapple to have any possible effect, you would need to eat between seven and ten whole fresh pineapples at one sitting. Tinned pineapple and pineapple juice contain little or no bromelain.

The final strategy, eating curry, has the greatest potential for getting things moving, but only if it is so hot that it causes discomfort and acts as a strong laxative. Then it could have the same effect as castor oil, which has been used for centuries to kick-start labour. It is thought that when the gut is stimulated, it in turn stimulates the uterus to cramp and spasm, thereby bringing on labour. Castor oil contains ricinoleic acid, or ricinic acid, which irritates the small intestine and has a strong laxative effect. One American study found that after a 60ml dose, 58% of women started labour within 24 hours, compared with just 4% of untreated women. However, this was just a small study, and self-treatment is not recommended. Castor oil can result in severe nausea and cramps, persistent diarrhoea, dehydration and other complications. If you want to try castor oil or an extremely hot curry, it is important to talk to a doctor or midwife first. They will be able to advise you according to your medical history, the position of your baby and the condition of your cervix.

There are other non-dietary strategies that might help and are less likely to have unpleasant side-effects, including sex, nipple stimulation or an alternative therapy such as homeopathy or acupuncture.

11 Breastfeeding – the best diet for you and your baby

Just because your baby has been born, it doesn't mean you can stop thinking about healthy eating. Even if you've chosen not to breastfeed or it hasn't been possible, a balanced diet is still important to help your body recover from all the work it's been doing and replenish the nutrient stores lost during pregnancy. If you are breastfeeding, this is even more important, as the food you eat will affect the growth and development of your baby. Also, before you know it, your little one will be eating proper food, and if you have good eating habits now, there's a much better chance that he or she will follow suit. Although weaning is a while off yet, you might want to start having conversations with your partner and any concerned relatives about what your baby is going to eat. Talking to them about your own beliefs about vegetarianism and your nutritional knowledge can be a good start.

If you found it hard to resist the temptations of ripe Brie or fried eggs while you were pregnant, the good news is that these can go back on the menu. However, small amounts of what you eat and drink will pass into your breast milk, so caffeine and alcohol should still be limited.

Breastfeeding gives your baby the best possible start in life. In the short-term it reduces the chances of your baby being hospitalised for diarrhoea or breathing problems, but the benefits to health stretch into adulthood. By paying a little extra attention to your diet, you can improve your baby's chances of a healthy future even more. It may even be possible to boost brain and eye development and reduce the risk of allergies and asthma.

Benefits of breastfeeding your baby

- Protection again vomiting, diarrhoea and constipation.
- Protection against ear infections.
- Protection against respiratory tract infections.
- A reduced risk of obesity and type 2 diabetes in later life.
- A reduced risk of allergies such as asthma and eczema.

What's in breast milk?

The composition of breast milk changes in the first few days after birth from colostrum, which is rich in protein and protective factors, to mature milk. It also changes during each feed from fore milk, which is more watery, to hind milk, which contains more calories and nutrients. It even varies with the time of day and with the weather, so your baby gets more fluids when it's hot, and really does get just what he or she needs.

On average, breast milk contains about 70kcal per 100ml. It is 1.3% protein, 4.1% fat and 7.2% carbohydrate and has a range of vitamins and minerals. In addition to providing nutrition, breast milk contains growth factors, hormones and other special proteins, antibodies, white blood cells and nucleotides, which help protect against infection.

How your diet affects your milk

Some components of breast milk are affected by the food you eat. The protein and carbohydrate content doesn't seem to vary, but studies have shown fat content can be altered. If you have a low-fat diet and low fat stores, the amount of fat in your breast milk is reduced. The levels of different fatty acids can also be altered. Women who eat more butter have higher levels of saturated fat in their breast milk, and women on macrobiotic diets have lower than average levels of saturated fat. In addition, women who consume more of the long-chain omega 3s DHA and EPA have more of these fatty acids in their milk. The breast milk of lacto-ovo-vegetarians contains more ALA (a short-chain omega 3) but less DHA (a long-chain omega 3) than that of meat-eaters. Vegans' breast milk has even more ALA and less DHA than that of lacto-ovo-vegetarians. It is also known that three-month-old babies breastfed by vegan mothers have around a third the amount of DHA in their blood compared to babies of meat-eaters. There is no evidence of health or developmental problems caused by vegans' lower DHA levels, but there hasn't been much research into it. Some experts argue that long-chain omega 3s are vital in the diets of breastfeeding mothers, and including some in your diet or taking supplements should be considered (see page 130).

There have been a small number of cases of vitamin B_{12} deficiency in babies of vegan mothers with low intakes of the vitamin and low levels in their breast milk. Deficiency results in megaloblastic anaemia and symptoms such as weakness, refusal to eat and delayed development. Most of the cases have involved babies who have been exclusively breastfed for up to 10 months to a year. A recent case, however, involved a five-month-old Italian boy who was admitted to hospital with severe growth and developmental problems and an enlarged liver and spleen. He was vitamin

B_{12} and iron deficient, and although his mother had taken multivitamin and vitamin supplements during pregnancy, she had stopped when he was born. Mild vitamin B_{12} deficiency in breastfed babies can be treated by giving the mother a supplement, but the Italian boy needed injections as he was severely deficient. These raised the level of vitamin B_{12} in his blood, but seven months later he still showed developmental delays. The supplements this vegan woman took contained 2.5µg vitamin B_{12} and it may be that a higher dose would have given her son larger vitamin B_{12} stores at birth. Lacto-ovo-vegetarians usually have higher intakes than vegans, but levels of vitamin B_{12} in breast milk have been found to be lower among lacto-ovo-vegetarians than among meat-eaters, and it is important for all vegetarians to be vigilant about this while breastfeeding.

As milk is rich in calcium, you may worry about getting enough calcium for your body to make breast milk. However, it has been found that breast milk calcium levels are fairly stable, irrespective of a mother's calcium intake. Research with macrobiotic women with very low calcium intakes found they had normal levels in their breast milk. Nevertheless, following pregnancy you will have less calcium in your body than normal, no matter how well you ate during pregnancy. Also, your body may be producing calcium-rich milk at the expense of your own needs. This could mean poor future bone health if you aren't careful. Calcium requirements increase from 700mg to 1250mg per day for breastfeeding, so it's a good idea to check you're eating enough calcium-rich foods to meet these high requirements (see page 118). If you're not, then it's best to take a supplement. Although calcium levels in breast milk are fairly stable, vitamin D levels are lower if mothers have lower levels, and this could affect calcium absorption. Vegetarians have been found to have lower vitamin D levels in winter and spring, and all breastfeeding women are advised to take a supplement.

The myth of poor-quality milk

Women sometimes believe their milk isn't very good. They may even be told they have 'poor-quality milk'. In reality, the composition of breast milk is unlikely to vary enough to affect your baby's feeding pattern or immediate growth, unless you are severely malnourished. It is much more likely that your baby's positioning and attachment while feeding need attention. If you are concerned about your milk supply and are thinking about giving your baby the odd bottle or switching to formula completely, don't rush into it. Make sure you first talk to your midwife or health visitor or call one of the breastfeeding helplines (see Resources). They should be able to offer you plenty of advice on establishing good breastfeeding.

Yummy – garlic milk

The foods, spices and drinks you consume while breastfeeding directly affect the flavour and odour of the milk you produce. You might think that garlic-flavoured milk would put a baby off feeding, but this doesn't seem to be the case. It is known that garlic transfers into breast milk – the odour has been detected by scientists, who report that it is at its strongest two hours after garlic is eaten – but babies seem to like it. In fact, babies have been found to stay at the breast longer, suck more often and consume more milk when their mother has eaten garlic.

Another great advantage of flavoured breast milk is that it prepares babies for weaning and enjoying a varied diet in later life. Breastfed babies are less likely to become fussy eaters. A greater acceptance of different flavours is apparent right from the beginning. A number of studies have found that babies exposed to certain flavours while breastfeeding, including garlic and aniseed, are more likely to enjoy the taste later when they are weaned.

A healthy diet for breastfeeding

A healthy vegetarian diet while you breastfeed is similar to that for any stage of life. However, there are some things you need to pay particular attention to. When you've just had a baby, it can be nice to have things laid down as simply as possible, so the guidelines below should help:

- At least **five portions of a variety of fruit and vegetables** every day. Fruit such as bananas and raisins are especially handy when you're busy with a new baby.
- **Protein foods**, such as eggs, cheese, nuts, seeds, beans and lentils.
- **Starchy foods**, such as bread, pasta, rice and potatoes. The extra energy you need for breastfeeding should come from having more of these foods rather than from snacks that are high in sugar or fat.
- **High-fibre foods**, such as high-fibre breakfast cereal and wholemeal bread and pulses. These are particularly important in the early days when constipation is a common problem.
- **Dairy foods**, such as milk and yogurt, or **dairy alternatives** with added calcium and vitamins B_{12} and D.
- **Omega 3-rich foods**, such as walnuts, are good, but long-chain omega 3s, such as DHA, are particularly important (see page 130).
- **Iron-rich foods**. During the last trimester of pregnancy, your baby accumulated most of the iron he or she needed, at the expense of your iron needs. Your iron levels may therefore have been depleted. You will also have

lost some blood when your baby was delivered, so it is important to replenish your iron levels now.

- **Plenty of fluids**. The general advice for people who are not breastfeeding is to drink at least six to eight glasses of fluid a day (approximately 1.2 litres). As you are likely to be producing about 800ml of milk a day, you obviously need more than this. However, there is no need to force yourself to drink more than you want. The best drinks are water, milk (skimmed, 1% or semi-skimmed), a fortified milk-alternative or pure fruit juice.

Ten tips for eating well with a new baby

When you have a new baby to look after, it can be difficult to think about your own diet. However, it is important to make healthy eating and regular meals a priority. This will benefit both you and your baby.

1 Always have healthy snacks at hand so that you don't have to rely on biscuits for an energy boost when you're busy.
2 Don't get into the habit of eating unhealthy take-aways and convenience foods because you're too tired to cook. Instead, keep meals simple. Buy ready-chopped vegetables for a stir-fry or try one of the almost instant meals listed here.
3 Have a big glass of water nearby every time you sit down to breastfeed. When you have a cup of tea or coffee, try to match it with a glass of water.
4 If your baby has a morning nap, make yourself a big sandwich with plenty of salad and put it in the fridge for later.

5 When things are going well and you have time to cook, try making extra to go in the freezer.

6 Shop online to make life easier. Stock up on staples such as pasta, couscous, rice and tins of chopped tomatoes, chickpeas and other legumes. And don't forget food for when you're too tired to cook, like baked beans, tinned soup and dried fruit, nuts and seeds.

7 Remember that eating well is more important now than how tidy your house is.

8 Try not to graze. Regular eating is important, but it is easy to get into bad habits when you are at home all day, which can result in weight problems.

9 When someone asks how they can help, ask them to cook a healthy meal, or suggest visitors bring fruit instead of chocolates sometimes.

10 Think about whether you are turning to food when what you really want is more sleep, fresh air, a bit of 'me-time' or emotional support. If you need help, ask for it (see Resources).

Ten almost-instant meals for busy mums

1 A jacket potato with baked beans and cheese, and a glass of orange juice.

2 Reduced-fat Cheddar or vegan cheese and tomato on toast.

3 A bowl of cereal with chopped banana or strawberries.

4 Greek salad in wholemeal pitta.

5 A peanut butter (or almond butter) and grated carrot sandwich.

6 Lentil soup and a granary roll.

7 Houmous with veg sticks and bread.

8 Toast with scrambled egg or scrambled tofu.

9 A falafel and salad wrap.

10 Pasta mixed with a jar of ragu and a tin of mixed beans.

Do you still need supplements?

Women who are breastfeeding are advised to take a supplement containing 10µg (400i.u.) of vitamin D every day. This is due to the re-emergence of rickets in recent years and is particularly important for vegetarians, as both vegans and lacto-ovo-vegetarians have been found to have lower than average vitamin D levels in their blood. If you were taking iron supplements during pregnancy because of anaemia then it's a good idea to continue for at least the first six weeks after delivery. Extra iron is also a good idea if you lost more than 400–500ml of blood during labour (which will be in your notes) or if you had heavy bleeding afterwards. If you're not sure whether your diet is supplying everything you need, particularly calcium and vitamin B_{12}, then a multivitamin and mineral supplement containing these nutrients is also a good idea. You may also want to take a DHA supplement.

Weight loss

It is important to take a balanced and sensible approach to weight loss when you've had a baby. It is not a good idea to lose 4 stones in four months, as some actresses reportedly do. Equally, you can't expect breastfeeding to make the pounds melt away if you eat chocolate biscuits by the packet.

Many new mums feel enormous pressure to lose weight after seeing pictures of super-slim celebrity mums. If you have a nanny, a personal trainer and your own chef, you may be able to follow in their footsteps; however, this isn't a recipe for successful breastfeeding or bonding with and enjoying your new baby. Trying to lose weight rapidly will also leave you feeling drained of energy and could mean both you and your baby miss out on vital nutrients.

It is estimated that breastfeeding requires about 500kcal per day. You probably need to double this for twins. During pregnancy, fat stores are laid down to supply some of the extra calories needed for breastfeeding, and the amount of food you need now will depend on how much fat you have stored. If you are thin, it's important to make sure you consume plenty of extra calories. You should make regular meals and snacks a priority and choose more energy- and nutrient-dense foods (see page 55). However, if you're overweight then it's important to get the nutrients you need by eating healthily (see page 170), while limiting your intake of high-sugar and high-fat foods.

If you have a very low-calorie diet, your milk supply will be affected. However, if you are overweight then slow weight loss won't adversely affect your milk supply. Research has shown that losing 1–2lb a week, through healthy eating and regular exercise, doesn't affect the amount or quality of a woman's breast milk, nor the amount of weight her baby gains. Some women find that breastfeeding makes them hungrier, but eating more low-GI foods can help with this. If you're struggling ask your health visitor or your doctor for more advice.

Foods to avoid when you're breastfeeding

There aren't any foods that you need to avoid completely while breastfeeding, but the following should be consumed in limited amounts:

- Try not to have too much **caffeine**. You may feel in need of a strong cup of coffee if you haven't slept well, but caffeine passes into breast milk, so it won't just be you who enjoys the stimulant effect. Also, babies can't metabolise caffeine as easily as adults, so it can build up in a baby's nervous system. There are no specific recommendations for breastfeeding, but following the guidelines for pregnancy would be sensible.

- **Alcohol** intake should be limited as, like caffeine, it passes into breast milk. It is recommended that you don't have more than one or two units once or twice a week. You may have heard that alcohol, particularly beer, is good for breastfeeding, but research has shown this is a myth. It was tested with two groups of mums in Pennsylvania, USA. The first had normal beer and the second non-alcoholic beer. Over the next four hours, the babies in both groups spent about the same amount of time feeding, while the mothers said they had experienced a normal letdown of milk and their babies had fed enough. However, weighing the babies afterwards revealed they consumed significantly less milk when their mothers drank alcoholic beer. In another study, babies were found to suck 15% more but get 30% less milk after their mums drank one to two units of alcohol. It could be that alcohol affects the mother's milk letdown (release of milk to the nipple area), so babies have to work harder.

  Curiously, babies don't seem to be put off by the smell or flavour of alcohol in their milk, which seems to be strongest 30 minutes to an hour after drinking. Babies given expressed milk from a bottle consume just as much when it contains alcohol as when it doesn't. In the long term, having the odd drink is unlikely to affect milk intake, as babies seem to compensate to some extent by drinking more later on. However, drinking alcohol while breastfeeding can have other effects. Alcohol may make mothers feel sleepy, but it actually makes babies more restless and spend less time in 'active sleep'. Also, in the long term it can affect a baby's well-being. Regular drinking (one or more units per day) has been found to adversely affect a baby's motor development.

- Some herbs are traditionally thought to dry up a woman's milk supply and, although these haven't been tested scientifically, it might be best to avoid taking large doses of sage, mint or parsley. Use in normal cooking is fine.

In the past, women with a family history of allergies were advised to avoid eating peanuts while breastfeeding, but this is no longer considered necessary. It was thought that peanut traces could pass into breast milk and increase a baby's allergy risk. However, recent studies have shown this is not the case and there is some evidence that early exposure to peanuts may even be beneficial.

Planning a night out

If you are going out for a drink, it is best to plan your feeding beforehand. Alcohol clears from your breast milk at about the same rate as from your blood (just over two hours per unit). However, this varies slightly according to your weight. For example, if a 9-stone woman drank six units of alcohol, it would take about 14 hours to clear from her milk, whereas an 11-stone woman would clear the same amount in about 13 hours.

The level of alcohol in your milk isn't affected by feeding, so 'pumping and dumping' is unnecessary. It is best to express enough milk before you start drinking to last your baby until the alcohol has completely left your system.

Women are sometimes advised to avoid orange juice, garlic, spicy meals or other foods while breastfeeding. Although certain foods affect individual babies, there is no need to limit your diet 'just in case'. It is better to eat as normal and keep an eye out for possible reactions to food, which might include general upset or restlessness, a rash, runny nose, wind, diarrhoea or explosive nappies.

If your baby has green bits in their nappy, it is probably not because of anything you or your baby has eaten. More likely, your baby has not been getting enough of the nutrient-rich hind milk that comes later during a feed, after the watery fore milk. This happens if the baby is switched from one breast to the other before having a chance to get the good stuff. If you're worried about the contents of your baby's nappies, talk to your midwife or health visitor.

If you suspect something in your diet is causing problems for your baby, then you could try cutting out a particular food for a week before trying it again. If you see a clear connection, then it may be best to steer clear of that particular food. However, it is important that you don't cut out whole food groups such as dairy or wheat unless you are completely confident your nutritional needs are still being met. There are many other reasons why babies suffer from problems such as eczema, diarrhoea and discomfort. Before changing your diet drastically it is best to talk to your doctor.

Colic

It can be very distressing if your baby has colic, and you are probably willing to give anything a go. However, before you cut anything out of your diet, it is important to know the facts. Sometimes improvements in your baby's feeding position can make a real difference. Although feeding may not be enjoyable or relaxing, it should be reassuring to know that babies with colic generally take just as much milk as others and gain weight normally. There has been some suggestion that babies of vegetarians are more likely to have colic, but this hasn't been tested specifically. It is speculation based on Dutch research which found that low vitamin B_{12} levels in early pregnancy were associated with more crying and colicky symptoms in babies. The media interpreted this to mean that eating steak in pregnancy leads to more contented babies.

What is colic?
Colic is thought to affect about one in five babies. It is characterised by periods of frantic crying at roughly the same time every day, typically early evening. A baby with colic may draw their knees up to their chest, pass wind and become red in the face. Colic generally appears in the first few weeks and disappears by the time a baby is three or four months old. If you are unsure whether your baby has colic, talk to your doctor to rule out other possible causes of distress.

Colic and cows' milk

In some babies, colic may be the result of lactose intolerance or an allergy to cows' milk. These may sound very similar, but they have quite different causes and should be treated differently.

Lactose intolerance

This is a sensitivity to the sugar (lactose) found in milk, including formula and breast milk. If a baby doesn't produce enough of the enzyme lactase, he or she is unable to break down the lactose sugar in the small intestine. The lactose therefore passes into the large intestine, where it ferments, producing hydrogen and methane gases and discomfort. If your baby is receiving formula, your health visitor may suggest switching to a lactose-free formula. Breast milk contains lactose no matter what you eat, so cutting out milk and dairy foods from your diet won't help: your body will still produce lactose for your milk. What you can do, however, is to give your baby lactase, for example Colief. This shouldn't be given to your baby directly but added to a small amount of expressed milk. Your baby can then be given this mixture from a spoon or cup, before being put to the breast as normal for a feed. The problem is often called 'transient lactose intolerance' because babies usually grow out of it. Once your baby is three to four months old, he or she should be producing sufficient lactase, so you won't need to supply it.

Cows' milk allergy

This is an immunological response to the proteins that cows' milk contains. These are found in most formula milks, as these are based on cows' milk, and in breast milk if the mother consumes milk or any milk products. If your baby is receiving any formula, then switch to a hypoallergenic variety. The only way to ensure your baby does not receive any cows' milk proteins from your breast milk is to remove all cows' milk and milk products from your diet. Your doctor or health visitor should be able to advise you on how to do this and how and when to try reintroduction. Allergies to cows' milk are rare and occur in only 0.5% of exclusively breastfed babies. Removing cows' milk for a week should be sufficient to see if this is the real cause.

Other causes and cures

Both lactose intolerance and cows' milk allergy are rare, and in most cases of colic the cause is unknown. Some research suggests that the baby's immature digestive tract could have difficulty coping with milk; as a result, the baby suffers from cramps. Colic may also be due to babies swallowing air bubbles when they feed or cry. To help minimise this, try to sit your baby as upright as possible during feeding, rather than laying him or her on their back, and burp your baby well. The drug simeticone may also help; this is an anti-flatulent, which changes small bubbles of gas into larger bubbles that are easier to burp up. Simeticone has been used for years and is readily available from pharmacists, for example as Infacol. It may also help if you feed at one breast until your baby has definitely had enough. Switching before your baby has had sufficient of the high-fat hind milk may mean that he or she feeds more to compensate, resulting in a larger volume of milk to cope with and more lactose than he or she can handle comfortably.

If you think something in your diet is triggering colic, it may be worth cutting out a particular food for a week to see if it makes any difference. The foods most commonly suspected of causing or aggravating colic include:

- tea and coffee;
- alcohol;
- cruciferous vegetables such as broccoli, cauliflower and cabbage: these may encourage the production of wind;
- wheat and corn;
- fish;
- eggs;
- onions;
- chocolate;
- citrus fruit.

Knowledge about colic is continually developing, so it is best to talk to your GP, health visitor or a registered dietitian. Be careful about using alternative treatments, as some, such as dicyloverine and star anise, have been found to be potentially dangerous. Sometimes women find breast-feeding a colicky baby so stressful they wonder if they would be better off with a bottle. However, formula-fed babies are much more likely to get colic than those who are exclusively breastfed.

Looking after yourself

New mums sometimes forget how important their own well-being is, but it's important to think about yourself as well as your baby. Eating well while you're breastfeeding is just as important for your own health as for your baby's. If your diet is less than ideal, you could suffer, even if your baby is fine. Research has shown that mothers can have signs of malnutrition, including bone demineralisation, B vita-min deficiencies and multiple infections, even when their baby appears to be healthy and has a normal or low-normal weight. So, by all means congratulate yourself if your baby is thriving, but remember this isn't everything. On the plus side breastfeeding also gives you certain benefits. It reduces your risks of breast cancer, ovarian cancer and osteoporosis.

Eating well while you're breastfeeding will boost your energy levels and could even help with postnatal depression. Although there is not much research into diet and postnatal depression, having a good intake of iron, zinc and vitamin B_6 are thought to be important. In addition, intakes of DHA and EPA are thought to affect mental health. Several studies have looked at whether intakes of these long-chain omega 3s can prevent or treat postnatal depression, but the results are inconclusive, with only some studies finding a benefit. However, given the other potential benefits of omega 3s, it's worth ensuring you have a good intake. Some herbal remedies that are believed to help improve mood, such as St John's Wort, are not recommended, as they may not be safe for babies. If you're not feeling yourself, then don't suffer in silence, as there is plenty of help available (see Resources).

Resources

Allergy UK

Medical charity dealing with allergy, food intolerance and chemical sensitivity.

www.allergyuk.org
Helpline: 01322 619 898

Association of Breastfeeding Mothers

Counselling hotline plus information about local breastfeeding clinics, support groups and baby cafés.

www.abm.me.uk
Helpline: 0300 330 5453 (9.30am to 10.30pm)

Breastfeeding Network (BfN)

Drop-in clinics plus help and support by phone and email.

www.breastfeedingnetwork.org.uk
Helplines: 0300 100 0210 or 0300 100 0212
Drugline: 0844 412 4665 (for information about taking prescription drugs)

Cry-sis

Support for families with excessively crying, sleepless and demanding babies.

www.cry-sis.org.uk
Helpline: 08451 228 669 (9am to 10pm)

Diabetes UK

Information and advice for diabetics and those with gestational diabetes.

www.diabetes.org.uk
Careline: 08451 202 960 (9am to 5pm Monday to Friday)

Healthy Start

Government scheme providing free supplements and food vouchers for pregnant women and new mums on a low income.

www.healthystart.nhs.uk

La Leche League

Local support groups and helpline with calls taken by mothers in their homes.

www.laleche.org.uk
Breastfeeding helpline: 08451 202 918

NCT (formerly National Childbirth Trust)

Organises antenatal classes and provides advice and support for pregnancy and early childhood. Will help put you in touch with other mums in your local area.

www.nct.org.uk

Helpline: 0300 330 0700 (9am to 7pm Monday, Wednesday, Thursday and Friday; 9am to 6pm Tuesday; Breastfeeding line [option 1] 8am to midnight every day)

NHS Direct

24-hour nurse advice and health information service. Lots of useful information on the website about pregnancy, breast-feeding and general health.

www.nhsdirect.nhs.uk
Information line: 0845 4647 or 111 (24 hours a day)

Tamba (Twins and Multiple Births Association)

Information and support network for parents of multiples.

www.tamba.org.uk
Twinline: freephone 0800 138 0509 (10am to 1pm and 7pm to 10pm every day)

Samaritans

Confidential emotional support, 24 hours a day.

www.samaritans.org
Tel: 08457 909090

Single Parent Action Network (SPAN)

National multi-racial organisation run by single parents working to improve the conditions of life for one-parent families in the UK and Europe.

http://spanuk.org.uk/
Tel: 0117 955 0860
Email: info@spanuk.org.uk

Tommy's

Advice and information, including free books and leaflets about pre-pregnancy and pregnancy.

www.tommys.org
Pregnancy line: 0800 0147 800 (9am to 5pm Monday to Friday to talk to a midwife)

Vegan Society

Guidance on well-planned vegan diets for parenthood.

www.vegansociety.com
Tel: 0121 523 1730 (9am to 5pm Monday to Friday)

Vegetarian Society

Information, advice and recipes for vegetarians.

www.vegsoc.org
Tel: 0161 925 2000 (8.30am to 5pm Monday to Friday)

Index